V-Shape Bichannel Spinal Endoscopy: Technique and Practice

Shisheng HE
(Edited by)

SCIENCE PRESS

Beijing

Responsible Editor: Mei Li

Copyright © 2023 by Science Press.
Published by Science Press.
16 Donghuangchenggen North Street
Beijing 100717, China.
Printed in Beijing.
All rights reserved. No part of this publication may be reproduced, stored in a retrieval system, or transmitted in any form or by any means, electronic, mechanical, photocopying, recording or otherwise, without the prior written permission of the copyright owner.

ISBN 978-7-03-075818-7

Contributors

Editor in chief
Shisheng He

Deputy editor in chief
Haijian Ni

Assistant editor in chief
Yunshan Fan

Section editors
Bo Wang, The First Affiliated Hospital of Dalian Medical University

Kaiming Wang, Bengbu Third People's Hospital

Chuanfeng Wang, Tenth People's Hospital of Tongji University

Zhongliang Deng, The Second Affiliated Hospital of Chongqing Medical University

Ziquan Shen, Bengbu First People's Hospital

Sheng Shi, Tenth People's Hospital of Tongji University

Chun Feng, Shanghai First Rehabilitation Hospital

Peitai Liu, Bengbu First People's Hospital

Huang Yan, Tenth People's Hospital of Tongji University

Ning Yan, Tenth People's Hospital of Tongji University

Xun Yang, Tenth People's Hospital of Tongji University

Qun Yang, The First Affiliated Hospital of Dalian Medical University

Deshun Yang, Nanjing Pukou Hospital of Traditional Chinese Medicine

Xin Zhang, Shanghai First Rehabilitation Hospital

Jia Chen, Tenth People's Hospital of Tongji University

Fangjing Chen, Tenth People's Hospital of Tongji University

Chengpei Zhou, Tangdu Hospital of Air Force Military Medical University

Yingchuan Zhao, Tenth People's Hospital of Tongji University

Shisheng He, Tenth People's Hospital of Tongji University

Zhengjian Yan, The Second Affiliated Hospital of Chongqing Medical University

Jixian Qian, Tangdu Hospital of Air Force Military Medical University

Guangfei Gu, Tenth People's Hospital of Tongji University

Haijian Ni, Tenth People's Hospital of Tongji University

Liang Cheng, The Third Affiliated Hospital of Southern Medical University

Shunzhi Yu, Tenth People's Hospital of Tongji University

Yunshan Fan, Tenth People's Hospital of Tongji University

Qingchu Li, The Third Affiliated Hospital of Southern Medical University

Amanda Ferland, Shanghai First Rehabilitation Hospital

Translators

Chaobo Feng, Guoxin Fan, Haoyu Gong, Xiaofei Guan, Xinbo Wu, Yanjie Zhu, Zhi Zhou, Zifei Zhou.

All translators are from Tenth People's Hospital of Tongji University.

Foreword

Over the last two decades, spinal endoscopy technology has led to the rapid development of minimally invasive spinal surgery, and various technologies and tools are emerging one after another. Looking back on the development of spinal endoscopy, from the arthroscopic to the thoracoscopic and laparoscopic, from microscope to microendoscopy, from uniportal and unichannel coaxial spinal endoscopy to biportal noncoaxial spinal endoscopy, from simple spinal endoscopy to high-definition, 4K and 3D digital spinal endoscopy, these technological advances have greatly expanded the indications from the lumbar spine to cervical and thoracic spine and promoted the development of modern minimally invasive spinal surgery technology. Spinal endoscopic surgery is no longer a "new" surgery based on the concept of interventional surgery, but takes spinal endoscopy as a tool to complete traditional spinal surgery with less trauma.

Under this background, Professor Shisheng He's team and Guanlong Company have developed the V-shape Bichannel Endoscopy (VBE) after five years, which is different from any existing endoscope in clinics. VBE is a brand-new uniportal bichannel endoscope and an original product independently developed by the Chinese people. The system can safely and efficiently complete lumbar decompression and interbody fusion via transforaminal approach under real-time and whole process endoscopic monitoring. It has two working modes of water medium and air medium so that spine surgeons can complete the operation under a familiar approach and visual situation, so as to reduce the learning curve.

This book is edited by Professor Shisheng He and well written by many minimally invasive spine surgery experts. It describes in detail the design principle, instrument composition, indications, surgical procedures, and surgical skills of the V-shape bichannel endoscopy, and provides a large number of case data and example pictures to enable readers to understand this new spinal endoscopy system, to better apply it to clinics and benefit patients. It is hoped that this book will be beneficial to those who are committed to spinal endoscopy.

Yue Zhou, MD
Director of Orthopedics Department of Chongqing Xinqiao Hospital
President of the International Society for Minimally Invasive Spinal Surgery
(ISMISS)
August 2021, Chongqing

Preface

As a representative key technology of spinal minimally invasive surgery, the development of spinal endoscopy lags behind arthroscopy. Because the object of operation for spinal endoscopy is the spine and the nerves, there are higher requirements for safety. Arthroscopic technology has been relatively secure since the 1970s because it is performed in the joint cavity with a high level of safety. However, in the early 1980s, doctors began to try to observe and operate on the spinal column with the help of arthroscopic instruments and technology.

The earliest spinal endoscopy technology was used to observe and operate through bilateral incisions, with the arthroscopy on the one side and instruments on the other side. In the middle and late 1990s, the third generation of spinal endoscopy, specifically the YESS endoscopy, developed rapidly. It integrated the light source, operation channel, observation endoscopy and flushing hole of spinal endoscopy, so as to make spinal endoscopy more minimally invasive and specific. In the last 20 years, this uniportal, unichannel coaxial spinal endoscopy had become the mainstream. It showed great advantages in simple discectomy and lateral stenosis decompression, and had achieved good results. As this uniportal and unichannel coaxial spinal endoscopy technology was more and more widely used, doctors had accumulated more and more experience. They were more and more aware of the advantages of spinal endoscopy technology. At this time, more doctors were not satisfied with the idea that spinal endoscopy technology was only applied to decompression of intervertebral disc herniation and lateral spinal canal stenosis; they hoped to use spinal endoscopy to complete more complex spinal operations, such as spinal fusion, osteophyte resection and decompression etc. At this time, this uniportal unichannel coaxial spinal endoscopy had encountered many problems: limited flexibility, low efficiency, time consumption, easy damage of instruments, etc.

We began to think about this problem in 2016 and wondered whether we could learn from the concept of arthroscopy to design a new spinal endoscope, increase the flexibility of spinal endoscope by increasing and expanding the working channel, and use bigger instruments, so as to improve the operation efficiency of spinal endoscope, reduce the damage of instruments and save costs. Under the guidance of this concept, we designed the V-shape Bichannel Endoscopy (VBE) system, together with Shandong Guanlong Medical Supplies Co., Ltd. In the past five years, with the support of experts in Shanghai, Guangzhou and the entire country of China, after more than ten versions of instrument improvement, many cadaver simulation operations and clinical verification, the finalization of design and naming were completed on June 18, 2020. The first VBE Lumbar Fusion Technology Seminar was held in December 2020. In April 2021, the Spinal Endoscopic Fusion Summit Forum and the Second VBE Lumbar Fusion Technology Symposium were organized, with more than 6000 online and offline participants. In April 2021, the clinical research paper on the application of the VBE system for intervertebral foraminoplasty was accepted by the *Journal of Orthopedic Surgery*. In April 2021, the clinical research applied to endoscopic decompression and interbody fusion was presented at the 20th Annual Meeting of the Pacific and Asian Society of the Minimally Invasive Spine Surgery (PASMISS) in the form of a speech, and was accepted as a speech at the 2021 Annual Meeting of the International Society for the Study of the Lumbar Spine (ISSLS). At present, VBE technology has been clinically applied in dozens of hospitals in China, achieved good results and attracted extensive attention.

VBE technology is different from the current UBE technology. The UBE technology uses the principle of arthroscopic operation and adopts two incisions. The working channel and endoscopic channel are separated and operated like arthroscopy. VBE technology integrates the working channel and endoscopic channel, which is a whole entity, and presents a "V" shape from the side view, so it is called V-shape Bichannel Endoscopy (VBE). It only needs one incision. The positions of instruments and endoscopes are fixed, making it easy to identify the position during operation and not lose direction. Therefore, it is a kind of endoscope completely different from UBE and represents different operation concepts. It is an original innovation. VBE can be operated in both air medium and water medium, and it is the first endoscopic system in the world that can be operated in both air medium and water medium. When the flushing water is turned off, it works like MED. When the flushing water is turned on, it is the transforaminal endoscope in water medium. Therefore, the operation is more convenient, and the doctors adapt more easily.

With the support of many experts in China and other countries, VBE, as a new type of spinal endoscopy, will be more widely used, gradually improved and developed. Its efficacy will also be verified by more practices. We expect VBE technology to benefit more patients in the future.

Shisheng He, MD
Director of Orthopedics Department of Tenth People's Hospital of Tongji University
August 2021, Shanghai

Contents

Chapter 1

Brief History of Spinal Endoscopic Surgery 1
1.1 History and Development of Unichannel Spinal Endoscopy 1
1.2 History of MED Technique 7
1.3 History of Bichannel Spinal Endoscopy 8

Chapter 2

Principles of V-Shape Bichannel Endoscopy System Design...................... 15
2.1 Keypoints of V-Shape Bichannel Endoscopy System Design 18
2.2 Composition of V-Shape Bichannel Endoscopy System 19
    2.2.1 V-Shape Channels 19
    2.2.2 Spinal Endoscope 21
    2.2.3 The Use of Trephine 21
    2.2.4 The Lengthened Surgical Instruments 23
    2.2.5 The Water Plugs 24
    2.2.6 The Choice of Interbody Fusion Cages................................... 24
    2.2.7 Bone Graft Materials and Biological Factors 26
2.3 Foraminoplasty and Working Cannula Placement.............................. 26
2.4 Comparison of V-Shape Bichannel Endoscopy System and Conventional Unichannel Spinal Endoscopy Techniques 27
2.5 Comparison of V-Shape Bichannel Endoscopic Fusion and Unichannel Spinal Endoscopic Fusion 28
2.6 Comparison of V-Shape Bichannel Endoscopy System and Unilateral Biportal Endoscopy Techniques 29

Chapter 3

Clinical Applied Anatomy for V-Shape Bichannel Endoscopy 31
3.1 General Anatomy of the Lumbosacral Spine...................................... 31
    3.1.1 Bone Structures of the Lumbosacral Spine 31
    3.1.2 Connections Between Vertebrae 33
    3.1.3 The Spinal Cord and Nerves of the Lumbosacral Spine 35
    3.1.4 The Vascular Distribution in the Lumbosacral Spine 36
3.2 Anatomy Related to V-Shape Bichannel Endoscopy Surgical Approaches 39
    3.2.1 Anatomy of the Lumbar Intervertebral Foramen 39
    3.2.2 Anatomy of the Lumbar Facet Joint 42
    3.2.3 The Safety Triangle 43

Chapter 4

V-Shape Bichannel Endoscopy Assisted Discectomy and Decompression 45
4.1 Application of Type I V-Shape Bichannel Endoscopy Decompression Cannula
 in Lumbar Surgery 46
    4.1.1 Structure of Type I VBE Decompression Cannula 46
    4.1.2 Indications 47
    4.1.3 Instruments 47
    4.1.4 Position 47
    4.1.5 Planning 47
    4.1.6 Anesthesia 48
    4.1.7 Establishment of Working Channel for Unichannel Endoscope
  System 48
    4.1.8 Establishment of Working Channel for Type I VBE Decompression
  Cannula 48
    4.1.9 Foraminoplasty with Type I VBE Decompression Cannula 49
    4.1.10 Discectomy and Decompression 50
4.2 Application of Type II V-Shape Bichannel Endoscopy Decompression Cannula
 in Lumbar Surgery 51
    4.2.1 Structure of Type II VBE Decompression Cannula 51
    4.2.2 Indications 51
    4.2.3 Instruments 52
    4.2.4 Position 52
    4.2.5 Planning 52
    4.2.6 Anesthesia 52
    4.2.7 The Establishment of the Working Cannula 53
    4.2.8 Discectomy and Decompression 53

Chapter 5

V-Shape Bichannel Endoscopic Lumbar Fusion 55
5.1 Anatomy 56
5.2 Surgical Instruments and Equipment 57
5.3 Layout of Operating Room 58
5.4 Surgical Indications 59
5.5 Surgical Contraindications 59
5.6 Surgical Methods 59
    5.6.1 Preoperative Preparation and Planning 59
    5.6.2 Body Position and Surface Location 60
    5.6.3 Operation Process 62
5.7 Precautions for Operation 71
    5.7.1 Preoperative Imaging Data Analysis and Surgical Planning 71
    5.7.2 Direction of Puncture 71
    5.7.3 Location of Working Cannula 71
    5.7.4 How to Use a Trephine to Remove Bones? 72

	5.7.5	Hemostasis	72
	5.7.6	To Ensure the Fusion of Bone Graft...	72
	5.7.7	Use of Water Plug	72
	5.7.8	Precautions of Decompression	73
	5.7.9	Management of Working Cannula Shift	73
	5.7.10	Avoidance of Vascular Injury	73
5.8	Postoperative Treatment		73
5.9	Prevention of Complications...		73
	5.9.1	Stimulation and Injury of the Outlet Root................................	73
	5.9.2	Injury of Exiting Root and Dural Sac	74
	5.9.3	Injury of Vessels and Organs in Front of Vertebral	74
	5.9.4	Malposition of Interbody Fusion Cage	74
	5.9.5	Nonunion of Bone Graft	74

Chapter 6

Clinical Application of V-Shape Bichannel Endoscopy 77
6.1   Application of V-Shape Bichannel Endoscopy in Lumbar Decompression 77
6.2   Application of V-Shape Bichannel Endoscopy in Lumbar Fusion 83
      6.2.1   VBE Lumbar Fusion for Lumbar Spinal Stenosis 83
      6.2.2   VBE Lumbar Fusion for Spondylolisthesis 99
6.3   VBE Lumbar Fusion for Lumbar Instability 107
6.4   VBE Lumbar Fusion for Recurrent Lumbar Disc Herniation 110

Chapter 7

Lumbar Surgery Rehabilitation 118
7.1   Introduction 118
7.2   Low Back Pain Clinical Practice Guideline 119
7.3   Preoperative Rehabilitation 121
7.4   Patient Education 125
7.5   Surgical Complications 125
7.6   Postoperative Evaluation 127
7.7   Postoperative Rehabilitation Principles 127
7.8   Postoperative Rehabilitation Protocols... 130

List of Abbreviations

ADL	Activities of Daily Living
AMD	Arthroscopic Microdiscectomy
AOPT	Academy of Orthopaedic Physical Therapy
BMP	Bone Morphogenetic Protein
CPK	Creatine Phosphokinase
CRP	C-Reactive Protein
CT	Computed Tomography
IDET	Intradiscal Electrothermal Therapy
IED	Irrigation Endoscopic Discectomy
ISSLS	International Society for the Study of the Lumbar Spine
LBP	Low Back Pain
MD	Microdiscectomy
MED	Microendoscopic Discectomy
METRx	Minimal Exposure Tubular Retractor
MIS-TLIF	Minimally Invasive Transforaminal Lumbar Interbody Fusion
MRI	Magnetic Resonance Imaging
MRN	Magnetic Resonance Neurography
OLIF	Oblique Lumbar Interbody Fusion
PASMISS	Pacific and Asian Society of the Minimally Invasive Spine Surgery
PBED	Percutaneous Biportal Endoscopic Decompression
PEID	Percutaneous Endoscopic Interlaminar Discectomy
PELD	Percutaneous Endoscopic Lumbar Discectomy
PETD	Percutaneous Endoscopic Transforaminal Discectomy
PE-TLIF	Percutaneous Endoscopic Transforaminal Lumbar Interbody Fusion
ROM	Range of Motion
SIJ	Sacroiliac Joint
SLR	Straight Leg Raise
STM	Soft Tissue Mobilization
TFSE	Transforaminal Spinal Endoscopy
THESSYS	Thomas Hoogland Endoscopic Spine System
TLIF	Transforaminal Lumbar Interbody Fusion
UBE	Unilateral Biportal Endoscopy
ULIF	Unilateral Biportal Endoscopic Lumbar Interbody Fusion
VBE	V-shape Bichannel Endoscopy
YESS	Yeung Endoscopic Spine System

Chapter 1

Brief History of Spinal Endoscopic Surgery

Section Editors:

Chuanfeng Wang, MD
Ning Yan, MD
Yingchuan Zhao, MD
Guangfei Gu, MD

    Because the working channel of spinal endoscopic surgery is established through the natural anatomical gaps and orifices, this kind of surgery causes little damage to the bone structure and soft tissue. Therefore, spinal endoscopic surgery is regarded as the minimally invasive spinal surgery in the defined sense. Patients will benefit from its merits, such as timely recovery. After decades of development, spinal endoscopy surgery has attracted more and more attention from specialists in spinal surgery, pain medicine, neurosurgery, and interventional radiology. Chinese traditional wisdom believes that: "With a mirror, people can dress up, with history as a mirror, we can know the rise and fall of dynasties; with people as a mirror, we can understand gains and losses." Hoping to give readers a better understanding, we briefly reviewed the history of spinal endoscopic surgery development.

1.1 History and Development of Unichannel Spinal Endoscopy

    In the 1940s, Valls J *et al.* began to try the posterolateral approach for lumbar spine surgery [1]. At that time, doctors mainly used puncture cannula to perform puncture biopsy on vertebral body tissue. In 1964, Lyman Smith first reported the use of papain for chemical lysis of the nucleus pulposus [2]. Under the guidance of X-ray, the intervertebral disc was punctured through the posterolateral approach of the lumbar spine. After the puncture needle reached the nucleus pulposus, papain was injected to dissolve and dehydrate the nucleus pulposus tissue, thereby achieving indirect decompression of the intervertebral disc, which is used to treat lumbar disc herniation. This was the first minimally invasive operation for lumbar disc disease. At present, this operation has been gradually eliminated due to various side effects, but the treatment of lumbar spine diseases through the posterolateral approach has been continuously developed and updated.

In 1973, Kambin used the Craig channel through the posterolateral approach to perform percutaneous aspiration of lumbar intervertebral disc under blind vision to treat encapsulated disc herniation and achieve the purpose of indirect decompression of the spinal canal [3]. In 1975, Japanese scholar Hijikata et al. introduced another non-direct vision percutaneous nucleotomy via the posterolateral approach [4]. The procedure was to introduce biopsy forceps into the intervertebral disc via a posterolateral approach, make a hole in the annulus to open a window, remove parts of the nucleus pulposus to reduce the pressure of the intervertebral disc, and relieve the stimulation of nerve roots and pain receptors around the intervertebral disc. In this way, the symptoms caused by disc herniation could be improved. This technique avoids the hemorrhage of the epidural venous plexus and the formation of secondary fibrous scars after surgery. Meanwhile, this surgical method causes little damage to the spine posterior structure and protects the spine stability. Therefore, the incidence of postoperative complications is lower than that of traditional open surgery and chemical lysis. Then in 1983, Kambin et al. developed a new surgical method [5]. They used a method similar to that of Hijikata to perform discectomy without visualization in 136 patients suffering from lumbar disc herniation and achieved a success rate of 72%. However, due to the larger diameter of the instruments used at that time, the incidence of nerve and blood vessel damage was kind of high. It is also difficult to treat L5/S1 intervertebral disc with this technique. In the same year, William Friedman reported the direct lateral approach of percutaneous suction of lumbar intervertebral disc, but this approach is prone to cause intestinal injury [6]. In 1985, Onik designed an automatic percutaneous intervertebral disc cutting and suction device that integrates cutting, washing, and suction [7]. Because this instrument has a smaller diameter, it significantly reduces complications such as nerve and blood vessel damage. In the same year, the American Academy of Orthopaedic Surgeons officially listed this method as one of the safe and effective methods for treating lumbar disc herniation, which greatly promoted the application of this surgery.

With the widespread use of arthroscopic equipment in joint surgery, Forst and Hausman first introduced arthroscopic equipment into spine surgery for the treatment of lumbar intervertebral discs disease in 1983 [8]. In 1988, Kambin described the arthroscopic imaging view of the protruding nucleus pulposus and annulus fibrosus tissue, and named this procedure arthroscopic microdiscectomy (AMD) [9]. In 1989, Schreiber et al. used indigo carmine staining to identify degenerative nucleus pulposus and annulus fibrosus fractures during surgery [10]. In 1990, Kambin described the concept of the safe triangle for the intervertebral foramina, which defined the exiting nerve root in the intervertebral foramen as the hypotenuse, the upper endplate of the lower vertebral body as the bottom edge, and the dura/traversing nerve root as the medial edge (Figure 1.1). Before this safe triangle concept, surgeons tended to use instruments with a small diameter to prevent iatrogenic nerve damage. Owing to this theory, surgeons have a better understanding of the anatomy of the intervertebral foramen, and this has made the application of large diameter instruments in endoscopic spinal surgery safer. More and more complex spine surgeries can be completed under the endoscope. The safe triangle concept provides theoretical foundation, and significantly promotes the development of endoscopic spinal surgery.

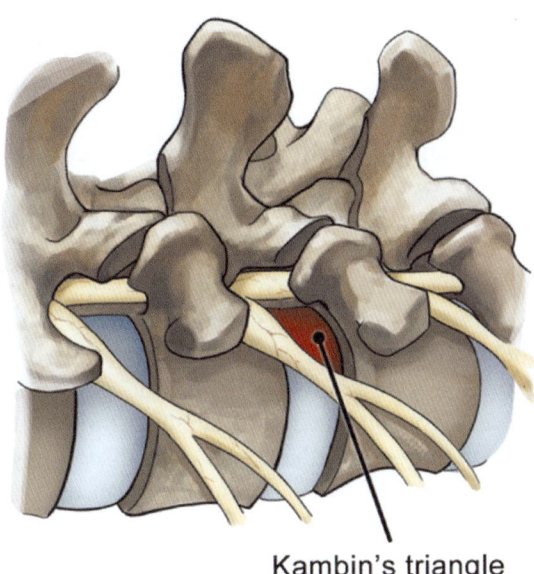

Kambin's triangle

FIG. 1.1 Kambin's triangle.

In 1993, Mayer *et al.* used an endoscope with a bevel angle to observe the rupture of fibrous annulus [11]. Mathews and Ditsworth described the foraminal approach in 1996 and 1998, respectively, which also opened the era of transforaminal spinal endoscopy (TFSE) surgery to treat lumbar disc herniation [12, 13]. Before this system, the endoscope used in spine surgery was similar to arthroscopy, requiring two channels for observation and operation separately, while the TFSE system allows the visualization and operation in a unichannel, and surgical instruments can be used in the working cannula flexibly in this system. Therefore, the TFSE can also reduce the damage to muscles and soft tissues caused by double channels. In 1997, Anthony Yeung designed a new generation of rigid, wide-angle, coaxial spine endoscopy system (Yeung Endoscopic Spine System, YESS), and also invented high-frequency radiofrequency electrodes [14, 15]. The YESS performs the nucleotomy through Kambin's triangle. This YESS greatly improves the accuracy and efficiency of transforaminal spine endoscopic discectomy. In 2001, Knight *et al.* tried to use lateral incision combined with holmium laser for foraminoplasty, and achieved satisfying results [16]. In 2002, Yeung and Tsou retrospectively analyzed 307 endoscopic discectomy cases, and found that the therapeutic effect was similar to that of traditional open surgery [17]. In the same year, Tsou and Yeung followed up 219 patients with non-encapsulated lumbar disc herniation who underwent transforaminal endoscopic surgery for at least one year. They concluded that the transforaminal endoscopic surgery is safe and effective to treat non-encapsulated lumbar disc herniation, and its clinical success rate is 91.2%.

In 2002, based on the YESS technique, Professor Thomas Hoogland creatively proposed the Thomas Hoogland endoscopic spine system (THESSYS) technique. THESSYS technique directly releases and decompresses the nerve root in the spinal canal through the intervertebral foramina. The THESSYS technique is widely accepted in the field. The key point of the THESSYS technique is to directly decompress the nerve structures by placing the working channel on the dorsal side of the spinal canal, according to the type of disc herniation. In order to place the working channel in the spinal canal ideally, foraminoplasty is usually required. Professor Hoogland designed different types of trephines and safe bone drills to expand the intervertebral foramen by removing the ventral part of the upper articular process. In 2005, Schubert and Hoogland reported the application of trephine for foraminoplasty during endoscopic surgery for patients with prolapsed lumbar disc herniation, with a success rate of 95.3%[18]. In the same year, Ruetten et al. introduced the concept of full endoscopy and reported the removal of the nucleus pulposus via the far lateral approach[20]. In 2006, Hoogland et al. published a prospective randomized controlled study of 280 consecutive patients with lumbar disc herniation[19]. Patients received endoscopic lumbar discectomy or endoscopic lumbar discectomy combined with intradiscal injection of low-dose (1000 U) chymotrypsin. The conclusion was that endoscopic discectomy with posterolateral approach could achieve satisfactory results in the treatment of lumbar disc herniation. Patients were more satisfied with the treatment of endoscopic discectomy combined with intradiscal injection of 1000 U of papaya chymotrypsin, and this method can be applied to any type of lumbar disc herniation, including the L5/S1 segment.

In 2006, Ruetten et al. reported the results of a 2-year follow-up of 331 patients with lumbar disc herniation who underwent translaminar approach endoscopic surgery[21]. The results showed that the leg pain of 82% of patients was significantly relieved, and 13% of patients had occasional leg pain after surgery. The result is similar to that of traditional surgery. However, this technique reduces the damage in the approach and the spinal canal, and reduces the formation of epidural scars. The recurrence rate of intervertebral disc herniation is 2.4%. No serious surgery-related complications occurred. The author believes that with appropriate surgical indications, the interlaminar approach has the advantage of minimally invasive surgery for the treatment of lumbar disc herniation. This technique is an effective and safe option for lumbar disc herniation. In addition, the interlaminar approach for the treatment of lumbar disc herniation is also a good supplement to the transforaminal approach.

In the same year, Choi et al. also reported the use of the interlaminar approach to treat 65 patients suffering from L5/S1 intervertebral disc herniation[22, 23]. All patients were followed up for more than one and a half years. The results showed that at the last follow-up, the leg pain VAS score and the lumbar ODI score were significantly improved, compared with their preoperative scores, and 90.8% of the patients were satisfied with the treatment effect. The average length of hospital stay was 12 hours, and the average time to return to work was 6.79 weeks. In their study, 2 patients had cerebrospinal fluid leakage, 9 patients had transient numbness after surgery, 1 patient had recurrence, and 2 patients were converted to open surgery; no infection was observed. They concluded that the percutaneous endoscopic translaminar approach is a safe and effective method for treating L5/S1 disc herniation, especially for patients who had difficulty in the transforaminal approach due to high iliac crest and other anatomical factors.

In 2007, Lee et al. performed endoscopic surgery on patients with lumbar disc herniation and disc migration [24]. According to the herniated disc migration direction and distance, it is concluded that the satisfaction rate of endoscopic surgery for patients with downward migration is 91.8%, and 88.9% for upward migration, 97.4% for mild migration, and 78.9% for high migration, and patients with highly migrated disc herniation need open surgery in some situations [25]. In 2007, Ruetten et al. reported 232 patients with lumbar disc herniation who underwent full endoscopic transforaminal lumbar discectomy, and found that minimally invasive endoscopic surgery can reach results similar to those of open surgery [26, 27]. It is worth noting that they used 4.2 mm working channel endoscopes and associated surgical instruments developed by their team.

With the vigorous development of endoscopy surgery, spinal endoscopy surgery has also received more and more attention from Chinese doctors. On October 15, 2003, the Minimally Invasive Spine Surgery Group of the Spinal Cord Injury Committee of the Chinese Society of Rehabilitation Medicine was formally established. Professor Shuxun Hou served as the first chairman, and Professor Yonglong Chi, Zhongjun Liu, and Guohua Lv served as vice-chairman. Many experts have emerged in the field of minimally invasive spine surgery in China, such as Professor Yue Zhou and Professor Xifeng Zhang. They have done a lot of pioneering work to promote the development of spinal endoscopy in China.

Since 2010, Professor Shisheng He started the standardized cadaver operation training for spinal endoscopy surgery in China. Therefore, many minimally invasive doctors have been trained, which has also promoted the vigorous development of spinal endoscopy surgery in China. After 2010, the spinal endoscopy in China ushered in a decade of rapid development. In 2015, hosted by the China International Exchange and Promotive Association for Medical and Health Care and undertaken by Shanghai Tenth People's Hospital, the Second China Spine Endoscopy Academic Conference was held. There were nearly 1000 registered participants, and many participants were willing to sit on the floor, just to be provided with an understanding of the most cutting-edge spinal endoscopy surgery (Figure 1.2). In the past 10 years, Chinese people have also put forward many original ideas or technologies based on their ingenuity, such as target technique, Beis technique, simplified technique, LiESS technique, ULESS technique, visualization technique, etc. At the same time, many versions of endoscopic equipment and tools have been invented and improved, so that spinal endoscopy has gradually developed from the previous simple decompression surgery to decompression and fusion surgery.

Endoscopic lumbar interbody fusion was first reported by Leu et al. in 1996, but this technique was not accepted widely at that time [28, 29]. It was not until 2013 that Jacquot et al. reported a clinical study of 57 patients undergoing transforaminal lumbar interbody fusion (TLIF) under full endoscopy [30]. However, symptomatic revision surgery due to cage migration was reported up to 22.8% of that time. The proportion of patients with poor results was up to 14%. They believed that endoscopic lumbar interbody fusion should not be recommended until the technique is mature. With the continuous improvement of surgery in endoscopic lumbar intervertebral disc removal and lumbar spinal canal decompression, the clinical efficacy improved continuously, and lumbar intervertebral body fusion surgery under full endoscopy has regained the attention of surgeons specializing in endoscopic spinal surgery [31–33].

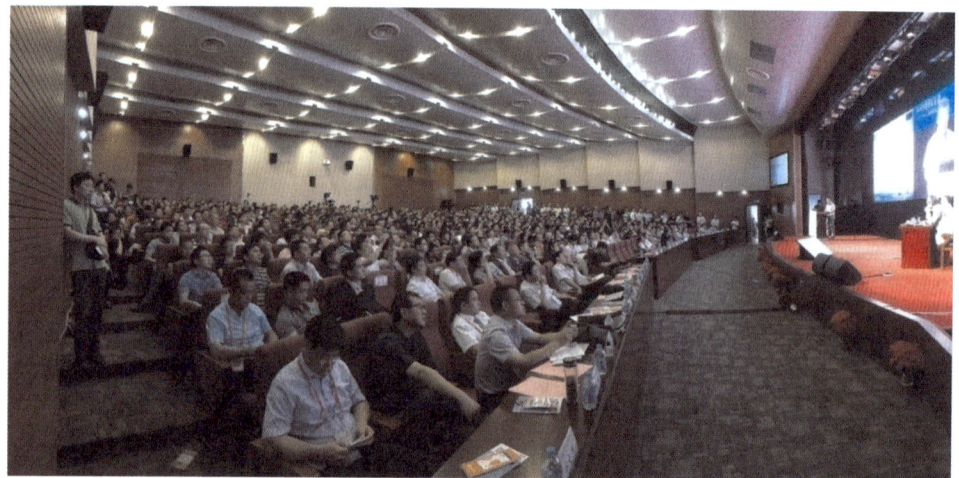

FIG. 1.2 Picture of the Second Academic Conference of China Spinal Endoscopy.

Nagahama *et al.* performed percutaneous endoscopic transforaminal lumbar interbody fusion (PE-TLIF) surgery on 25 patients with degenerative lumbar spondylolisthesis, and achieved satisfactory results [34]. They believed that PE-TLIF surgery is effective and feasible. However, they also pointed out that the surgeon must have good surgical skills, and the hospital should be equipped with nerve electrophysiological monitoring. Ahn et al. reviewed endoscopic lumbar fusion surgery in 2019, and pointed out that the current level of evidence for PE-TLIF surgery is low [35]. However, the concept and early results of endoscopic fusion are encouraging. PE-TLIF surgery has many limits, such as the high rate of potential complications, the difficulty of intervertebral space management and fusion cage migration, the limited source of bone graft materials, and the high radiation exposure.

In 2018, Professor Yue Zhou published their early cases of endoscopic interbody fusion under general anesthesia and nerve monitoring [36]. A total of 7 patients with single-segment lumbar spine diseases underwent endoscopic fusion surgery, and all patients were followed up for more than 2 years. The data showed that postoperative pain and function of the patients were significantly improved, and all patients achieved interbody fusion. However, the author pointed out that the current endoscopic fusion is still an immature surgery with high technical requirements, narrow indications, and a high rate of potential complications. Because of the small operating space, it is difficult to operate in the intervertebral space and implant the fusion cage. In addition, the incidence of exiting nerve root injury and cage migration is high; in addition, it also has a long learning curve and requires a wealth of experience in endoscopic operation.

Lastly, it also faces other problems, such as limited bone grafting and excessive radiation exposure.

Later in 2020, Professor Yue Zhou published a clinical study of endoscopic fusion with a larger sample size [37]. This article retrospectively analyzed the clinical data of 75 patients who underwent PE-TLIF or minimally invasive transforaminal lumbar interbody fusion (MIS-TLIF) from April to August 2018. There were 35 cases in the PE-TLIF group and 40 cases in the MIS-TLIF group. Their study found that the serum creatine kinase on the first day postoperatively and C-reactive protein on the third day postoperatively in the PE-TLIF group were significantly lower than those in the MIS-TLIF group. The total blood loss, intraoperative blood loss, and postoperative drainage in the PE-TLIF group were significantly reduced compared with the MIS-TLIF group. The VAS scores and ODI of low back pain and lower extremity pain were significantly improved in the two groups. There was no significant difference in the fusion rate between the PE-TLIF group and the MIS-TLIF group. They concluded that there was no significant difference in the short-term and medium-term results of the two types of surgery. Compared with MIS-TLIF, PE-TLIF showed advantages in surgical injury and postoperative pain. However, PE-TLIF has relatively limited indications and a long learning curve, which requires strict selection of patients. In the future, more high-quality clinical studies are needed to further verify the value of PE-TLIF.

In summary, the current endoscopic fusion technique still has certain limits: relatively complicated surgical procedure, long learning curve, high incidence of potential complications such as nerve injury and cage migration, incomplete visualization during operations such as dealing with intervertebral space and implantation of cages, insufficient bone graft materials and a large radiation exposure dose. However, with the development and improvement of endoscopic surgical instruments and the improvement of surgical skills, the future of full endoscopic lumbar interbody fusion is expected to be safer, produce less surgical complications, and provide better surgical efficacy and a higher rate of interbody fusion.

1.2 History of MED Technique

The surgical procedure of Microendoscopic Discectomy (MED) was first reported by Foley in 1997 [38]. In 1999, based on the original MED system, Medtronic Sofamor Danek USA developed the second-generation of MED system (Minimal Exposure Tubular Retractor, METRx). Compared with the MED system, the second-generation METRx system has significantly improved imaging, equipment, and operability. MED technique combines the advantages of the traditional posterior laminectomy technique and the minimally invasive technique under the endoscope. MED surgery establishes the surgical approach by gradually expanding the channel, and completes the laminectomy, facet joint resection, nerve root canal decompression, and intervertebral disc resection in the working channel. In the past, all these procedures could only be finished by open surgery.

MED surgery establishes a surgical approach by serial dilator, and completes all surgical operations in the working channel. Therefore, compared with traditional surgery, the MED surgery shows advantages like smaller incision, less paravertebral muscle damage, less intraoperative bleeding, and quicker postoperative recovery. Because the imaging system can enlarge the view of the operating field, the anatomical structure can be identified more clearly during the operation, and various operations can be completed more precisely. Therefore, MED can avoid the disadvantages of traditional surgery, such as massive damage to bone and soft tissue caused by poor surgical view and inaccurate operation. Compared with traditional surgery, MED surgery can greatly preserve the integrity of the posterior spine structure, and effectively reduce the probability of postoperative scar adhesion, spinal instability and adjacent vertebrae [39, 40].

MED surgery is not only suitable for discectomy, but also has obvious advantages in decompression for lumbar spinal stenosis, especially for severe lumbar spinal stenosis. The use of unilateral approach and bilateral decompression technique can not only complete spinal canal decompression, but also reduce surgical damage and bleeding, and maximize spine stability. Spinal fusion surgery with MED is very suitable for patients with spinal instability and lumbar spondylolisthesis. Of course, MED surgery also has certain limits. Firstly, MED system can only provide two-dimensional images, and the MED operation is performed through a channel under the air medium. Compared with water medium, the air medium has limits, such as relatively poor clarity due to bleeding, and the need to repeatedly wipe the lens during surgery. During the operation, muscles and other soft tissues can easily enter the channel, and it is usually disrupted to clean these muscles or other soft tissues. Cleaning the soft tissue will prolong the operation time and increase the complexity of the operation. In addition, MED surgery requires the surgeon to watch the monitor while performing the surgery, which also has a long learning curve.

1.3 History of Bichannel Spinal Endoscopy

The unichannel spinal endoscope system used in clinical practice integrates the perfusion channel, light source, and camera into one endoscope. It not only has the advantages of clear vision and less injury, but also obvious limits: the vision channel and the working channel are coaxial, the vision lacks a three-dimensional sense, the operation is not flexible enough and the space is limited. Generally, the working channel can only use one surgical instrument. Cooperation between multiple instruments in the working channel is impossible for the unichannel spinal endoscope system. Thus, the surgical efficiency is kind of low, and the application in complicated cases is limited. Additionally, surgeons often find themselves in the situations that the target can be viewed clearly, but is difficult to be reached through the unichannel endoscope system. Therefore, some scholars have begun to explore endoscopic spinal surgery like arthroscopic surgery, which can be completed under dual or even multiple channels. In this way, the system is more flexible and makes the working space larger. What is more, surgeons can complete complicated cases using multiple channels at the same time.

In fact, looking back on history, arthroscopic assisted spinal endoscopic surgery is the earliest two channel endoscopic surgery. Forst and Hausman used arthroscopic equipment to perform lumbar disc surgery as early as 1983 [8]. In 1988, Kambin described the arthroscopic view of the prominent nucleus pulposus and annulus fibrosus tissue [9]. Around the 1990s, Kambin et al. began to try the dual-channel method to assist in spine surgery [39]. The dual-channel technology at that time was a bilateral dual-channel technology, with one side of the spinous process as an observation channel and the other side as an operating channel. In 1996, De Antoni et al. also reported the application of two independent channels of observation, and operation for discectomy with the aid of arthroscopy, which greatly improved the flexibility and efficiency of the operation [41]. In 2001, Dr. Abdul Gaffar from Bahrain reported unilateral biportal endoscopy (UBE) technique at the annual meeting of the American Academy of Orthopaedic Surgeons, which attracted the attention of scholars. In 2003, South Korean neurosurgeon Jinhwa Eum also reported the UBE technique research at the 4th biennial meeting of Korea-Japan conference on spine surgery. However, with the vigorous development and improvement of MED technology and unichannel spine endoscopy technologies such as YESS and THESSYS, the dual-channel spine endoscopic technology seems to gradually fade out. Only a few doctors still insist on using this technique.

In recent years, with the development of the UBE theory and the optimization of related surgical instruments and technologies, dual-channel spinal endoscopic sur- gery has gradually been revived. Korean doctors like Dr. Eum and Dr. Son have made great contributions to the development of dual-channel spine endoscopy. They used the UBE technique for the interlaminar approach and the transforaminal approach. The indications include lumbar, cervical, and thoracic diseases. The establishment of a special UBE society has promoted the development of this technique worldwide. In 2013, Soliman reported the use of irrigation endoscopic discectomy (IED) for minimally invasive treatment of lumbar disc herniation, and patient satisfaction reached 95% at 12 months after surgery [42]. Later, he used IED surgery to perform endoscopic spinal decompression on patients with lumbar spinal stenosis [43]. The 28-month follow-up results showed that 87% of patients had satisfactory decompression results.

In 2016, Eum et al. used percutaneous biportal endoscopic decompression (PBED) for the decompression of lumbar spinal stenosis [44]. They found that this technique has a good surgical view, and can effectively decompress the central area of the spinal canal and lateral recess area through unilateral laminectomy. Compared with the decompression surgery under the microscope, PBED surgery not only avoids bilateral incisions, but also reduces surgical damage. In 2017, Park JH et al. first reported the use of the UBE surgery for cervical foramina and cervical disc removal [45]. Heo et al. also reported the use of the UBE technology for lumbar fusion surgery in the same year [46]. 69 patients with single-segment lumbar spine disease received lumbar fusion surgery using the UBE technique. All patients had satisfactory postoperative clinical effects, and the complication rate was 7.2%. However, the investigator did not report the rate for interbody fusion. In 2018, Kim and Choi reported that 14 patients underwent lumbar fusion using the UBE technology, and all patients achieved good results [47]. The authors also did not report the postoperative fusion rate.

In 2019, Heo et al. compared the outcomes of unichannel, dual-channel spinal endoscopy and microscopic minimally invasive surgery in the treatment of lumbar spinal stenosis [48]. The study concluded that all three surgical methods had achieved good results. The single/dual channel endoscopy group has the advantage of reducing immediate postoperative pain. It is an effective method to treat lumbar central spinal stenosis and can effectively replace traditional microscope decompression. In 2020, Park et al. randomly divided 64 patients with lumbar spinal stenosis into two groups, and underwent bilateral decompression surgery through unilateral approach using dual-channel or microscopic unilateral approach respectively [49]. The study found that there were no significant differences in the operation time, blood loss, postoperative complications, or the improvement of clinical symptoms one year after the operation between the two groups. This study suggested that the clinical results between dual-channel endoscopic spinal surgery and microscope assisted surgery in the treatment of lumbar spinal stenosis were similar. Another randomized controlled study also showed that dual-channel endoscopic spinal surgery is better than channel-assisted microscopic spinal canal decompression in the treatment of lumbar spinal stenosis [50]. Dual-channel endoscopic spinal surgery showed certain advantages, such as shortened operation time and hospital stay, less postoperative drainage and reduced dosage of postoperative opioids.

Recently, the dual-channel spinal endoscopy surgery has gradually attracted attention in China and been used by surgeons in treating degenerative spinal diseases. Tian et al. used the UBE technology to treat 25 cases of lumbar disc herniation and 26 cases of lumbar spinal stenosis [51]. Compared with preoperative symptoms, all patients had pain relief and function recovery, and the excellent-and-good rate at the last follow-up reached 96.1%. They concluded that the UBE technology has the characteristics of clear vision, large operating space, relatively simple surgical instrument requirements, convenience, and flexibility. The clinical effect in treating lumbar disc herniation and lumbar spinal stenosis is excellent. A meta-analysis conducted by Chinese scholars compared the dual-channel spine endoscopy technique with the microscope assisted minimally invasive technique [52]. The results showed that there were no significant differences between the two groups in operation time, complication rate, back pain, and leg pain VAS score or ODI score.

Compared with traditional open surgery, the UBE technique is a minimally invasive surgery. This operation enriches the minimally invasive surgical options of the spine and is also a good supplement to unichannel endoscopic spine technique. The UBE technique uses water medium, which has a clearer vision than MED surgery. The UBE technique is flexible with a large processing range. Traditional surgical instruments can be directly used in the UBE surgery and the UBE technique is very efficient in lamina decompression. For UBE assisted lumbar fusion surgery, the surgical field is very clear, and the decompression procedure is very precise. During the UBE surgery, the endoscope can be inserted into the intervertebral space, and the whole procedure can be clearly monitored. The operating channel of the UBE system allows the insertion of a fusion cage and a nerve retractor at the same time. Thus, the nerve root and dural sac can be protected to reduce the risk of nerve injury. In addition, the UBE technique is more similar to the traditional spine surgery, and the learning curve of this technique is relatively low for spine surgeons. The UBE surgery can use traditional surgical instruments and is relatively cheap. For hospitals with only arthroscopic equipment, this kind of minimally invasive spinal surgery can also be performed. At present, studies have proved that fluoroscopy during the UBE surgery is less than percutaneous endoscopic lumbar discectomy (PELD) surgery, and the surgeon and the patient will receive less radiation exposure.

The UBE technique also has certain limits. Compared with unichannel spinal endoscopic surgery, UBE requires two surgical incisions and cause more damage to soft tissues. The UBE surgery usually requires a drainage tube. It is reported that the incidence of dural sac tear can be as high as 13.2%. Once the dural sac tear occurs during UBE surgery, it might mean that the minimally invasive operation cannot be completed. In addition, the complications of UBE surgery should not be ignored. A study showed that 82 of 797 patients (10.29%) who accepted UBE surgery had postoperative complications [53]. The most common complications were epidural hematoma and incomplete nerve decompression (both were 18 cases, 2.26%). A total of 35 patients had to undergo a revision surgery, and 56 patients were hospitalized for observation for more than 2 weeks. Of course, the complication incidence is related with the learning curve. The first 50 patients undergoing UBE surgery have a higher complication possibility. In addition, compared with unichannel spine endoscopic technique, the UBE technique has no obvious advantage in discectomy [54-56]. The UBE technique is similar to the traditional laminectomy. It will cause more bone structure damage, resect the ligamentum flavum, stretch the dural sac, and increase the risk of postoperative sacr adhesions. Also, the UBE surgery generally requires general anesthesia. In addition, two radiofrequency electrodes are needed during the operation, which will increase the economic burden to the patient. Compared to lateral approach, the UBE technique shows little advantage in dealing with posterior revision surgery.

Because the application time of the UBE technique is relatively short, high-quality clinical research evidence is still lacking. Particularly, studies about UBE-assisted fusion surgery are few, with relative low quality, the analysis of complications and fusion rate is insufficient, and lack of long-term follow-up. Therefore, multi-center, large sample, long-term follow-up clinical studies and randomized controlled trials are needed to further verify the advantages and disadvantages of the UBE technique.

References

[1] Valls J., Ottolenghi C.E., Schajowicz F. (1948) Aspiration biopsy in diagnosis of lesions of vertebral bodies, *J. Am. Med. Assoc.* **136**, 376.
[2] Smith L. (1964) Enzyme dissolution of the nucleus pulposus in humans, *JAMA* **187**, 137.
[3] Kambin P., Ed. (1990) *Arthroscopic microdiscectomy: Minimal intervention spinal surgery.* Urban & Schwarzenburg, Baltimore, MD.
[4] Hijikata S., Yamagishi M., Nakayma T. (1975) Percutaneous discectomy: A new treatment method for lumbar disc herniation, *J. Todenhosp.* **5**, 5.
[5] Kambin P., Gellman H. (1983) Percutaneous lateral discectomy of the lumbar spine: A preliminary report **174**, 127.
[6] Friedman W.A. (1983) Percutaneous discectomy: An alternative to chemonucleolysis, *Neurosurgery* **13**(5), 542.
[7] Onik G., Helms C.A., Ginsberg L., *et al.* (1985) Percutaneous lumbar diskectomy using a new aspiration probe: Porcine and cadaver model, *Radiology* **155**(1), 251.
[8] Forst R., Hausmann B. (1983) Nucleoscopy – A new examination technique, *Arch. Orthop. Trauma Surg.* **101**(3), 219.
[9] Kambin P., Nixon J.E., Chait A., *et al.* (1988) Annular protrusion: Pathophysiology and

roentgenographic appearance, *Spine (Phila Pa 1976)* **13**(6), 671.
[10] Schreiber A., Suezawa Y., Leu H. (1989) Does percutaneous nucleotomy with discoscopy replace conventional discectomy? Eight years of experience and results in treatment of herniated lumbar disc, *Clin. Orthop. Relat. Res.* (238), 35.
[11] Mayer H.M., Brock M. (1993) Percutaneous endoscopic lumbar discectomy (PELD), *Neurosurg. Rev.* **16**(2), 115.
[12] Mathews H.H. (1996) Transforaminal endoscopic microdiscectomy, *Neurosurg. Clin. N. Am.* **7**(1), 59.
[13] Ditsworth D.A. (1998) Endoscopic transforaminal lumbar discectomy and reconfiguration: A postero-lateral approach into the spinal canal, *Surg. Neurol.* **49**(6), 588; discussion 597–598.
[14] Yeung A.T. (1999) Minimally invasive disc surgery with the Yeung Endoscopic Spine System (YESS), *Surg. Technol. Int.* **8**, 267.
[15] Tsou P.M., Yeung A.T. (2002) Transforaminal endoscopic decompression for radiculopathy secondary to intracanal noncontained lumbar disc herniations: Outcome and technique, *Spine J.* **2**(1), 41.
[16] Knight M.T., Ellison D.R., Goswami A., *et al.* (2001) Review of safety in endoscopic laser foraminoplasty for the management of back pain, *J. Clin. Laser Med. Surg.* **19**(3), 147.
[17] Yeung A.T., Tsou P.M. (2002) Posterolateral endoscopic excision for lumbar disc herniation: Surgical technique, outcome, and complications in 307 consecutive cases, *Spine (Phila Pa 1976)* **27**(7), 722.
[18] Schubert M., Hoogland T. (2005) Endoscopic transforaminal nucleotomy with foraminoplasty for lumbar disk herniation, *Oper. Orthop. Traumatol.* **17**(6), 641.
[19] Hoogland T., Schubert M., Miklitz B., *et al.* (2006) Transforaminal posterolateral endoscopic discectomy with or without the combination of a low-dose chymopapain: A prospective randomized study in 280 consecutive cases, *Spine (Phila Pa 1976)* **31**(24), E890.
[20] Ruetten S., Komp M., Godolias G. (2005) An extreme lateral access for the surgery of lumbar disc herniations inside the spinal canal using the full-endoscopic uniportal transforaminal approach-technique and prospective results of 463 patients, *Spine (Phila Pa 1976)* **30**(22), 2570.
[21] Ruetten S., Komp M., Godolias G. (2006) A new full-endoscopic technique for the interlaminar operation of lumbar disc herniations using 6-mm endoscopes: Prospective 2-year results of 331 patients, *Minim. Invasive Neurosurg.* **49**(2), 80.
[22] Choi G., Lee S.H., Raiturker P.P., *et al.* (2006) Percutaneous endoscopic interlaminar discectomy for intracanalicular disc herniations at L5-S1 using a rigid working channel endoscope, *Neurosurgery* **58**(1 Suppl): ONS59-68; discussion ONS59-68.
[23] Choi G., Lee S.H., Bhanot A., *et al.* (2007) Percutaneous endoscopic discectomy for extraforaminal lumbar disc herniations: Extraforaminal targeted fragmentectomy technique using working channel endoscope, *Spine (Phila Pa 1976)* **32**(2), E93.
[24] Lee S., Kim S.K., Lee S.H., *et al.* (2007) Percutaneous endoscopic lumbar discectomy for migrated disc herniation: Classification of disc migration and surgical approaches, *Eur. Spine J.* **16**(3), 431.
[25] Choi G., Lee S.H., Lokhande P., *et al.* (2008) Percutaneous endoscopic approach for highly migrated intracanal disc herniations by foraminoplastic technique using rigid working channel endoscope, *Spine (Phila Pa 1976)* **33**(15), E508.
[26] Ruetten S., Komp M., Merk H., *et al.* (2007) Use of newly developed instruments and endoscopes: Full-endoscopic resection of lumbar disc herniations via the interlaminar and lateral transforaminal approach, *J. Neurosurg. Spine* **6**(6), 521.
[27] Ruetten S., Komp M., Merk H., *et al.* (2008) Full-endoscopic interlaminar and transforaminal lumbar discectomy versus conventional microsurgical technique: A prospective, randomized, controlled study, *Spine (Phila Pa 1976)* **33**(9), 931.
[28] Leu H.F., Hauser R.K. (1996) Percutaneous endoscopic lumbar spine fusion, *Neurosurg. Clin. N. Am.* **7**(1), 107.
[29] Leu H.F., Hauser R.K., Schreiber A. (1997) Lumbar percutaneous endoscopic interbody fusion, *Clin. Orthop. Relat. Res.* (337), 58.
[30] Jacquot F., Gastambide D. (2013) Percutaneous endoscopic transforaminal lumbar interbody fusion: Is it worth it, *Int. Orthop.* **37**(8), 1507.

[31] Komp M., Hahn P., Oezdemir S., *et al.* (2015) Bilateral spinal decompression of lumbar central stenosis with the full-endoscopic interlaminar versus microsurgical laminotomy technique: A prospective, randomized, controlled study, *Pain Physician* **18**(1), 61.

[32] Li Z.Z., Hou S.X., Shang W.L., *et al.* (2017) Modified percutaneous lumbar foraminoplasty and percutaneous endoscopic lumbar discectomy: Instrument design, technique notes, and 5 years follow-up, *Pain Physician* **20**(1), E85.

[33] Li Z.Z., Hou S.X., Shang W.L., *et al.* (2016) Percutaneous lumbar foraminoplasty and percutaneous endoscopic lumbar decompression for lateral recess stenosis through transforaminal approach: Technique notes and 2 years follow-up, *Clin. Neurol. Neurosurg.* **143**, 90.

[34] Nagahama K., Ito M., Abe Y., *et al.* (2019) Early clinical results of percutaneous endoscopic transforaminal lumbar interbody fusion: A new modified technique for treating degenerative lumbar spondylolisthesis, *Spine Surg. Relat. Res.* **3**(4), 327.

[35] Ahn Y., Youn M.S., Heo D.H. (2019) Endoscopic transforaminal lumbar interbody fusion: A comprehensive review, *Expert Rev. Med. Devices* **16**(5), 373.

[36] Wu J., Liu H., Ao S., *et al.* (2018) Percutaneous endoscopic lumbar interbody fusion: Technical note and preliminary clinical experience with 2-year follow-up, *Biomed. Res. Int.* **2018**, 5806037.

[37] Ao S., Zheng W., Wu J., *et al.* (2020) Comparison of preliminary clinical outcomes between percutaneous endoscopic and minimally invasive transforaminal lumbar interbody fusion for lumbar degenerative diseases in a tertiary hospital: Is percutaneous endoscopic procedure superior to MIS-TLIF? A prospective cohort study, *Int. J. Surg.* **76**, 136.

[38] Foley K.T., Smith M.M., Rampersaud Y.R. (1999) Microendoscopic approach to far-lateral lumbar disc herniation, *Neurosurg. Focus* **7**(5), e5.

[39] Kambin P., Schaffer J.L. (1989) Percutaneous lumbar discectomy. Review of 100 patients and current practice, *Clin. Orthop. Relat. Res.* (238), 24.

[40] Kambin P., Casey K., O'Brien E., *et al.* (1996) Transforaminal arthroscopic decompression of lateral recess stenosis, *J. Neurosurg.* **84**(3), 462.

[41] De Antoni D.J., Claro M.L., Poehling G.G., *et al.* (1996) Translaminar lumbar epidural endoscopy: Anatomy, technique, and indications, *Arthroscopy* **12**(3), 330.

[42] Soliman H.M. (2013) Irrigation endoscopic discectomy: A novel percutaneous approach for lumbar disc prolapse, *Eur. Spine J.* **22**(5), 1037.

[43] Soliman H.M. (2015) Irrigation endoscopic decompressive laminotomy. A new endoscopic approach for spinal stenosis decompression, *Spine J.* **15**(10), 2282.

[44] Hwa Eum J., Hwa Heo D., Son S.K., *et al.* (2016) Percutaneous biportal endoscopic decompression for lumbar spinal stenosis: A technical note and preliminary clinical results, *J. Neurosurg. Spine* **24**(4), 602.

[45] Park J.H., Jun S.G., Jung J.T., *et al.* (2017) Posterior percutaneous endoscopic cervical foraminotomy and diskectomy with unilateral biportal endoscopy, *Orthopedics* **40**(5), e779.

[46] Heo D.H., Son S.K., Eum J.H., *et al.* (2017) Fully endoscopic lumbar interbody fusion using a percutaneous unilateral biportal endoscopic technique: Technical note and preliminary clinical results, *Neurosurg. Focus* **43**(2), E8.

[47] Kim J.E., Choi D.J. (2018) Biportal endoscopic transforaminal lumbar interbody fusion with arthroscopy, *Clin. Orthop. Surg.* **10**(2), 248.

[48] Heo D.H., Lee D.C., Park C.K. (2019) Comparative analysis of three types of minimally invasive decompressive surgery for lumbar central stenosis: Biportal endoscopy, uniportal endoscopy, and microsurgery, *Neurosurg. Focus* **46**(5), E9.

[49] Park S.M., Park J., Jang H.S., *et al.* (2020) Biportal endoscopic versus microscopic lumbar decompressive laminectomy in patients with spinal stenosis: A randomized controlled trial, *Spine J.* **20**(2), 156.

[50] Kang T., Park S.Y., Kang C.H., *et al.* (2019) Is biportal technique/endoscopic spinal surgery satisfactory for lumbar spinal stenosis patients?: A prospective randomized comparative study, *Medicine (Baltimore)* **98**(18), e15451.

[51] Tian D., Liu J., Zhu B., *et al.* (2020) Unilateral biportal endoscopic technique for lumbar disc herniation and lumbar spinal stenosis, *Chin. J. Orthop.* **40**(17), 1155.

[52] Chen T., Zhou G., Chen Z., *et al.* (2020) Biportal endoscopic decompression vs. microscopic

decompression for lumbar canal stenosis: A systematic review and meta-analysis, *Exp. Ther. Med.* **20**(3), 2743.

[53] Eun S.S., Eum J.H., Lee S.H., *et al.* (2017) Biportal endoscopic lumbar decompression for lumbar disk herniation and spinal canal stenosis: A technical note, *J. Neurol. Surg. A: Cent. Eur. Neurosurg.* **78**(4), 390.

[54] Lee H.G., Kang M.S., Kim S.Y., *et al.* (2020) Dural injury in unilateral biportal endoscopic spinal surgery, *Global Spine J.* 2192568220941446.

[55] Kim W., Kim S.K., Kang S.S., *et al.* (2020) Pooled analysis of unsuccessful percutaneous biportal endoscopic surgery outcomes from a multi-institutional retrospective cohort of 797 cases, *Acta Neurochir. (Wien)* **162**(2), 279.

[56] Park M.K., Park S.A., Son S.K., *et al.* (2019) Clinical and radiological outcomes of unilateral biportal endoscopic lumbar interbody fusion (ULIF) compared with conventional posterior lumbar interbody fusion (PLIF): 1-year follow-up, *Neurosurg. Rev.* **42**(3), 753.

Chapter 2

Principles of V-Shape Bichannel Endoscopy System Design

Section Editors:

Shisheng He, MD
Qingchu Li, MD
Liang Cheng, MD
Sheng Shi, MD

Since 1970s, the arthroscopic technology has made great progress and has been widely applied in joint surgery with the development of optics, electronics, and imaging technology. The arthroscopy, as a minimally invasive technique, is much easier to be applied and promoted because there is natural space with no important nerves and blood vessels in the articular cavity, which makes the operation relatively safe. In comparison, the development and application of the spinal endoscopy lag behind arthroscopy. The spine lacks anatomical cavities, and the spinal cord and cauda equina in the spinal canal are easily damaged, which will lead to a serious negative outcome, and requires a more sophisticated procedure during the spinal surgery. Consequently, it was not until the early 1980s that the surgeon began to apply endoscopic techniques to spinal surgery.

Arthroscopy, laparoscopy, and thoracoscopy are a multi-portal and multi-channel technology. The surgeon can establish multiple working channels at different incisions so that the surgical instruments and the endoscope can cooperate with each other, which makes the surgical procedures more convenient. Inspired by arthroscopic techniques, some surgeons began to employ two working channels to observe and remove the intervertebral disc in the early 1980s. In 1983, Forst and Hausmann used the modified arthroscopic technology to directly observe and remove herniated discs [1]. Specifically, they inserted an arthroscopic instrument on one side of the spine to observe the herniated disc, and inserted a surgical instrument on the other side to remove the herniated disc. However, the intraoperative observation and surgical procedures were very difficult, and the risk of neural injury was relatively high, even with repeated X-ray fluoroscopic monitoring. After that, some researchers still tried to use the bichannel spinal endoscopy to remove the discs, *e.g.*, Dr. Antoni from Argentina reported the anatomy, indications, and advantages of the unilateral bichannel spinal endoscopy techniques in 1996 [2].

In the late 1990s, the spinal endoscopy technology was rapidly developing. In order to reduce surgical trauma, Yeung designed the YESS spinal endoscopy system, which integrated camera, lavage, light source and instrument channels together [3]. Currently, this technology has been developed as the most commonly used uniportal and unichannel coaxial spinal endoscopy system. The biggest advantage of the YESS spinal endoscopy system is that the surgical trauma is small under an unnatural cavity. Compared with the knee articular cavity, the spine does not have natural cavities. Therefore, the spinal endoscope needs to insert working channel to avoid the surrounding soft tissues. The spinal endoscopy system applied to the thoracic and lumbar spine can provide illumination and clear vision, and magnify the anatomical structures of the surgical field. In the past 20 years, some operation techniques, such as foraminoplasty, extra-disc decompression technology, visualized trephine technique, have been widely applied. At the same time, the surgical instruments of spinal endoscopy system have also been greatly improved. These operation techniques and tools have strongly promoted the progress of percutaneous endoscopic lumbar discectomy. After that, the uniportal and unichannel coaxial spinal endoscopy technology, represented by YESS and TESSYS technology proposed by Yeung and Hoogland, has been widely used internationally. The classic open lumbar discectomy might result in the formation of epidural scar, of which 10% patients may become clinically symptomatic. However, percutaneous endoscopic transforaminal discectomy (PETD) techniques can protect the posterior ligaments and articular process, and therefore, reduce the incidence of postoperative lumbar spine instability, articular process hyperplasia and intervertebral space stenosis. Besides, the PETD will not affect the epidural vascular system, which may avoid chronic nerve ischemia and fibrosis. Therefore, the PETD techniques can significantly reduce the associated surgical complications. Currently, the uniportal and unichannel coaxial spinal endoscopy system has been widely applied in the discectomy and the treatment of lateral spinal stenosis, and the clinical outcomes have been confirmed by many clinical studies [4–10].

The uniportal and unichannel coaxial spinal endoscopy system has been welcomed by many surgeons and patients, due to less trauma, good curative effect, and fast recovery. With the advancement of spinal endoscopic technology and the improvement of the technical level of minimally invasive spine surgeons, more and more surgeons not only use the spinal endoscopic technology to remove the intervertebral discs and to treat the lateral spinal stenosis, but also expand the indications of spinal endoscopic technology to treat severe spinal stenosis and spinal fusion. In order to minimize surgical trauma, the surgical instrument and working channel of traditional spinal endoscopy system are relatively small, *e.g.*, the diameter of the most used working channel is 6.9 mm (YESS spinal endoscopy system) or 8 mm (Vertebris spinal endoscopy system), which result in a limited surgical field and a narrow movement range of the surgical instruments. Therefore, there are many problems when dealing with complex spinal diseases, including limited operative space, high probability of equipment damage, low efficiency, and long operative time. Although spinal surgery technology is constantly developing, the surgery goal remains the same: to optimize clinical efficacy and reduce the surgical trauma, which greatly inspires the development and improvement of all of these technologies.

The V-Shape Bichannel Endoscopy system (VBE) consists of two channels, the endoscopic channel and the working channel (Figure 2.1). The two channels converge at the front end at a certain angle, and the side view is in a "V" shape, so it is named as the

V-Shape Bichannel Endoscopy system. The two channels can cooperate with each other through one surgical incision. Therefore, the VBE system integrates the advantages of multi-portal endoscopy such as arthroscopy, laparoscopy and the uniportal unichannel coaxial spinal endoscopy system, and has the characteristics of minimally invasive and convenient operating. In addition, since the diameters of two working channels of the VBE system can be designed according to the needs of the operation, the working channels can be used compatibly with conventional spine endoscopes or the small diameter endoscope exclusively for the VBE system, so as to accomplish the operation with larger space on the backside, such as endoscopic fusion and posterior decompression (Figures 2.2 and 2.3). With two channels, the VBE system enables surgeons to complete surgical procedures through the working channel under monitoring through the endoscopy channel. Therefore, the VBE system can truly achieve visualized operation under full-time and real-time monitoring. The original design intention of the VBE system is to increase the flexibility of endoscopic operations, improve efficiency, and reduce costs, which can make up for shortcomings of the uniportal and unichannel coaxial spine endoscopy system. With these merits, the VBE system can expand the indications of spinal endoscopic surgery to complex spinal diseases, such as lumbar interbody fusion.

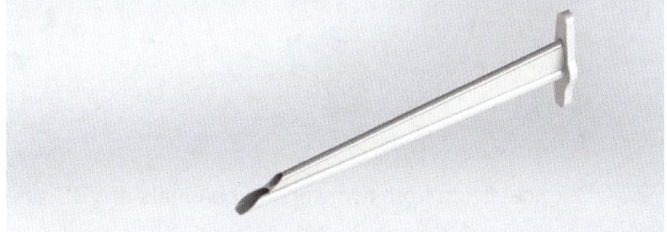

FIG. 2.1 Schematic diagram of VBE cannula.

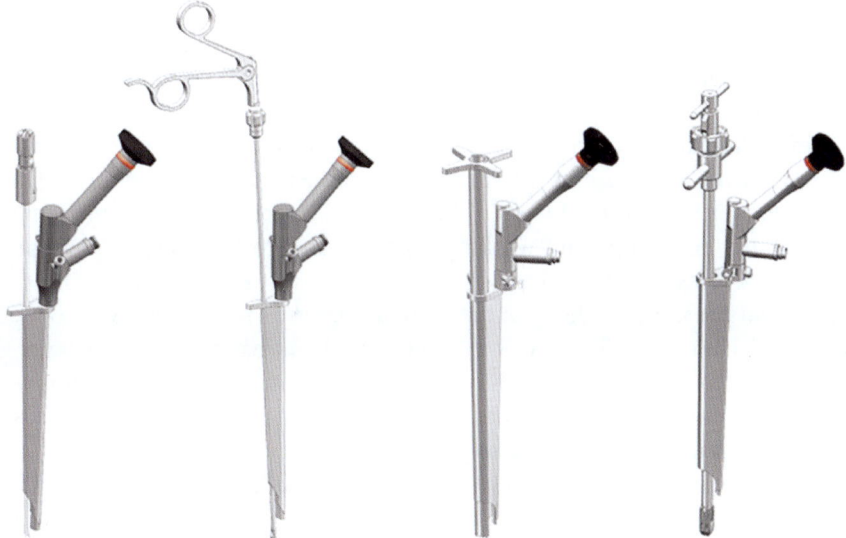

FIG. 2.2 Illustrations of the coordination between two working channels.

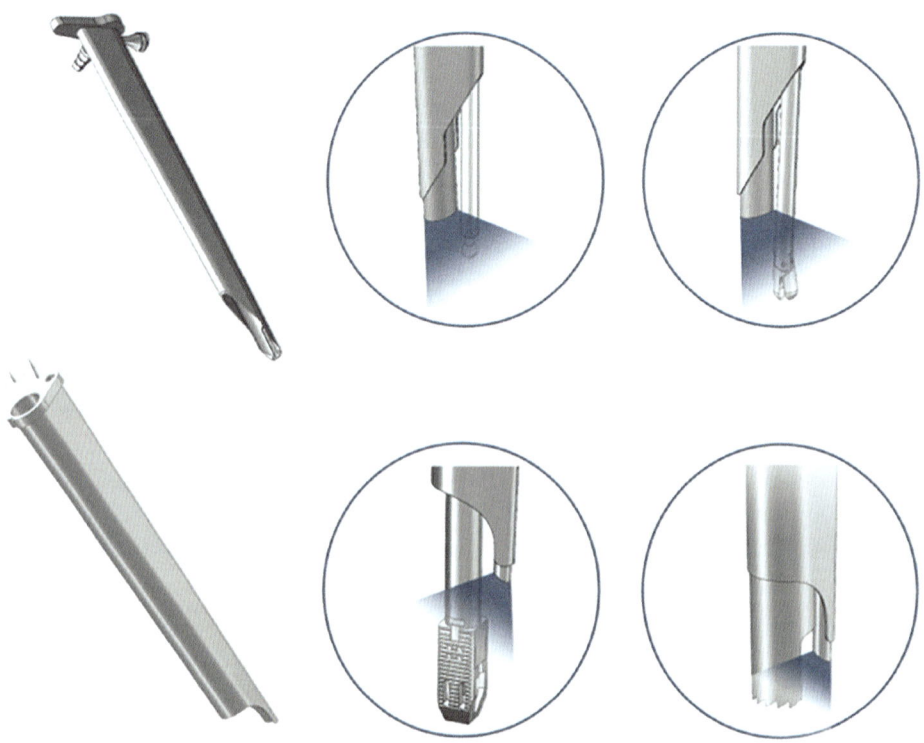

FIG. 2.3 Surgical fields from two working channels of VBE system.

2.1 Keypoints of V-Shape Bichannel Endoscopy System Design

The principal purposes of designing V-Shape Bichannel Endoscopy system are as follows.

(1) Since the current uniportal and unichannel coaxial spinal endoscopy system has only one working channel, all surgical procedures must be performed in this channel. Moreover, it is inflexible, and the operative space of surgical instruments is limited, since the endoscope and working channel need to be moved simultaneously during the procedures. Specifically, it is difficult for the surgical instruments to reach the area beyond the edge of the channel, which increases the difficulty of operation. Therefore, the VBE system is expected to have more working channels like arthroscopy and laparoscopy, to increase the working range of surgical instruments, to make the instruments and endoscopy cooperate with each other, and finally to increase the flexibility and the surgical view of the spine endoscope.

(2) The working channel diameter of traditional spine endoscopy is relatively small, and thus the matched instruments are also very tenuous and expensive, which leads to lower work efficiency. Moreover, the tenuous surgical instruments are easily

damaged, especially when dealing with bony lesions and complex lesions, which cause an increased surgical cost. Therefore, when designing the V-shape bichannel spine endoscopy, we expected that conventional spine surgical instruments can be applied to endoscopy, which will eventually improve surgery efficiency, shorten operation time, and decrease the probability of surgical instrument damage. As a result, the overall operation cost will be reduced since the cost of surgical instruments is lower.

(3) Endoscopic intervertebral fusion often requires inserting a fusion cage. In order to ensure the fusion cage implanted smoothly and safely without nerve injury, it requires the procedures be monitored under full-time and real-time visualization. However, the current unichannel spinal endoscopy system has not met the requirements, so another working channel should be added at this moment. With two channels, one used for real-time endoscopic monitoring and the other used for implanting a fusion cage, full-time and real-time visualization can be achieved, which will ensure the surgical safety and avoid the occurrence of nerve injury.

(4) For some difficult and complicated cases, such as intervertebral disc herniation with calcification, osteophytes on the posterior edge of the vertebral body, treating lesions with the VBE system and extended conventional surgical instruments will significantly increase surgical efficiency and achieve better clinical outcomes.

(5) The VBE system mainly works in the medium of water, but it can also work in the air medium like the microendoscopic discectomy. Therefore, the VBE is compatible with the microendoscopic discectomy, and is thought to provide unique advantages. Worldwide, the VBE system is the first type of the uniportal bichannel spinal endoscopy system that can be used both in air and water media.

(6) The VBE system is compatible with the traditional unichannel spinal endoscopy system. All of the surgical instruments and equipment of the unichannel spinal endoscopy system can be used in VBE, which is the supplement and development of the unichannel spinal endoscopy system. The unichannel endoscopy system can fully meet the requirements and achieve good outcomes when used for simple spinal degenerative diseases. However, when dealing with more complicated spinal diseases, which are difficult to treat using the unichannel spinal endoscopy system, the V-shape bichannel spine endoscopy system will play a better role. Therefore, VBE expands the indications of spine endoscopy.

2.2 Composition of V-Shape Bichannel Endoscopy System

2.2.1 V-Shape Channels

The two working channels are combined into a "V" shape as a whole to form a working cannula. The "V" shape design prevents the endoscope and the surgical tool from colliding with each other at the tail end, which ensures the surgical procedure goes smoothly. The working channel of VBE has its own water circulation system, including flushing holes and water outlet holes. The two working channels can be made into different diameters according to clinical needs, so the V-shape working channels for different purposes can be conveniently replaced during the operation. The most used working cannulas at present are as follows.

(1) The working cannula for decompression (Figures 2.4 and 2.5). The working cannula of VBE system consists of a large channel with an inner diameter of 6.5 mm and a small channel with an inner diameter of 3.8 mm. The working cannula is divided into two types according to the position of the large and small channels. The type I VBE working cannula consists of a small channel on the top and a large channel on the bottom. Specifically, the conventional spinal endoscopy can be used for observation through the large channel, while the surgical instruments such as drills, trephines and reamers can be used for foraminoplasty through the small channel. Conversely, the type II VBE working cannula consists of a large channel on the top and a small channel on the bottom. Specifically, the VBE customized small diameter endoscope can be used for observation through the small channel, while the surgical instruments can be used for performing the surgical procedures and decompression, such as removal of nucleus pulposus and foraminoplasty, through the large channel, which can improve surgical efficiency and decrease the probability of equipment damage.

(2) The working cannula for interbody fusion (Figure 2.6). The working cannula of the VBE system consists of a large working channel with an inner diameter of 13.1 mm on the top, and a small endoscopic channel with an inner diameter of 3.8 mm on the bottom. Specifically, the VBE customized small diameter endoscope can be used for observation through the small working channel, while the conventional surgical instruments for decompression, removal of nucleus pulposus, and fusion cage implantation can be used through the large working channel, which makes the surgical procedures more efficient.

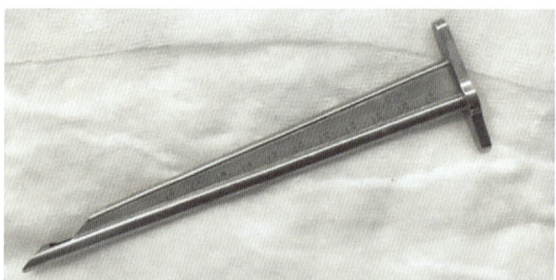

FIG. 2.4 Type I VBE working cannula for decompression.

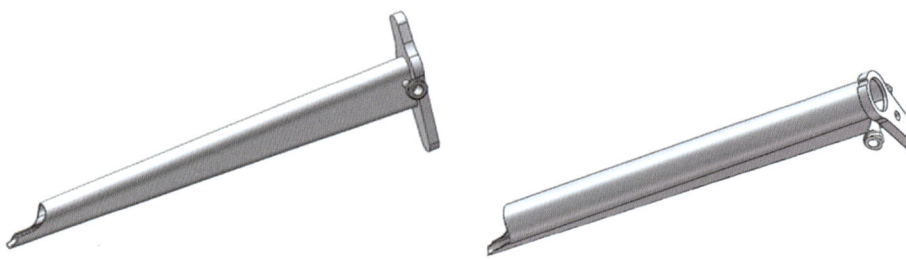

FIG. 2.5 Type II VBE working cannula for decompression.

FIG. 2.6 The VBE working cannula for interbody fusion.

2.2.2 Spinal Endoscope

The VBE system is designed with two types of spinal endoscopes. One is the most used uniportal and unichannel spinal endoscope, with an outer diameter of 6.3 mm (Figure 2.7), and the other is a spinal endoscope specially customized for the VBE system, with a small outer diameter of 3.6 mm (Figure 2.8), which can be alternately used. Moreover, because that the customized smaller diameter spinal endoscope and the other working channel of the VBE system are not coaxial, the relative position between the endoscope and the surgical instruments is adjustable, which can enlarge the surgical field and make the observation more convenient. The design concept of the VBE system is that the endoscope and the surgical instrument can be used alternately and cooperatively within the upper and lower different channels, which significantly increases the flexibility of the spinal endoscopy, and is especially convenient for the complex spinal diseases. In addition to the specially customized small diameter spinal endoscopy, the VBE system is also compatible with the endoscopic equipment and instruments from most manufacturers of the uniportal and unichannel spinal endoscopy, which may also cut down the cost.

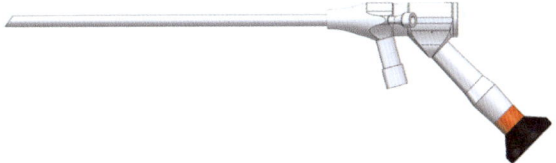

FIG. 2.7 The uniportal and unichannel spinal endoscope with an outer diameter of 6.3 mm.

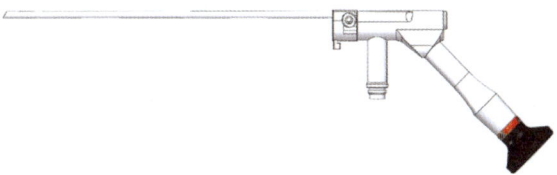

FIG. 2.8 Spinal endoscope with a small outer diameter of 3.6 mm.

2.2.3 The Use of Trephine

The V-shape bichannel endoscopy system has a series of specially designed matching trephines, which are used to safely remove the articular process during endoscopic interbody fusion. The matching trephines include ordinary trephine (Figure 2.9), bone-removal trephine with internal thread (Figure 2.10), bone-removal trephine with internal thread that can be tightened (Figure 2.11), and semi-trephine (Figure 2.12). The trephine has a scale, so the trephine depth can be observed under the monitor of the endoscopy to avoid neural damage, and to ensure the surgical safety. Specifically, the ordinary trephine is relatively thin and sharp and can be used to remove the articular process, while the trephine with internal thread is mainly used to remove the excised bone. During surgical procedures, we always first use the ordinary trephine, which is relatively thin and sharp, to resect the articular process to reach the required safe position and to shake the trephine to loosen or break the bone. Then, we use the trephine with internal thread to take out the excised or broken bone pieces. If the above procedures go smoothly, the sawn bone can be taken out completely through the internal thread, or else, we can use a trephine with internal thread that can be tightened to saw the articular process, and then to tighten the trephine to take out the bone pieces. Generally, we can take out most of the bone pieces through the above operations, and some small bone pieces can be taken out with nucleus pulposus forceps under the endoscopic monitoring. For some patients, the articular process, especially the superior articular process of the lower vertebral body, is very close to the posterior edge of the vertebral body. In order to avoid damaging the upper nerve roots, ordinary trephines and trephines with internal threads should not saw too deeply. After the sawn bone is taken out, we can use a semi-trephine to cut off the remaining upper articular process under endoscopic monitoring. During the operation, the serrated side of the semi-trephine should be placed at the caudal side to protect the upper nerve roots. Additionally, the rongeur forceps can be used to remove the articular process bone pieces to further reduce the risk of neural damage induced by the semi-trephine.

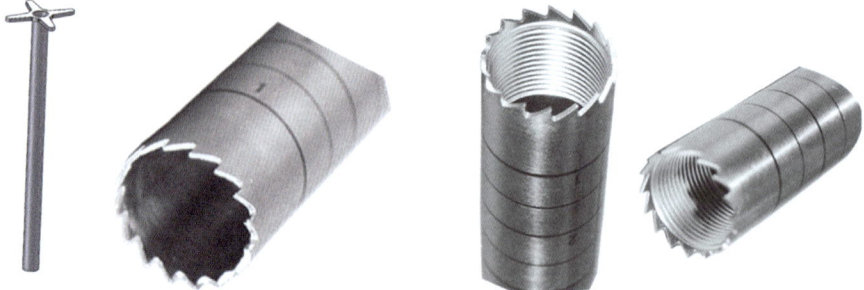

FIG. 2.9   Ordinary trephine.

FIG. 2.10   Bone-removal trephine with internal thread.

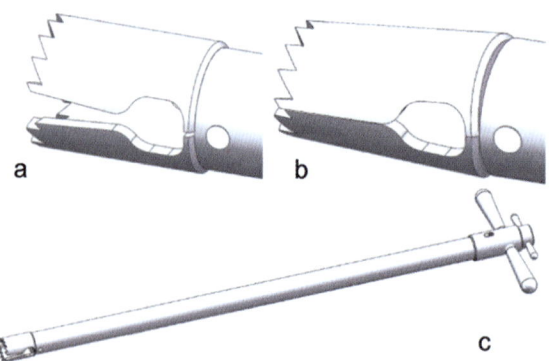

FIG. 2.11   Bone-removal trephine with internal thread that can be tightened.
(a) open status; (b) tightened status; (c) overall view of the trephine.

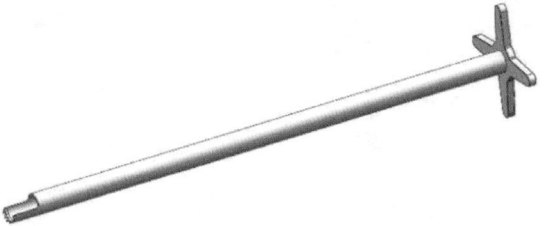

FIG. 2.12 Semi-trephine.

2.2.4 The Lengthened Surgical Instruments

During the process of endoscopic fusion, all traditional rongeur forceps, nucleus pulposus forceps, and instruments for the treatment of intervertebral spaces including spreaders, reamers, and spatulas can be used in the V-shape bichannel endoscopy system after being lengthened. Moreover, marking surgical instruments with scales at the distal and proximal ends can avoid entering the interbody space too deeply and damaging the surrounding important tissues (Figures 2.13 and 2.14). The diameter of the current surgical instruments for the spinal endoscopy is small, and the working efficiency is relatively low, so it takes a long time to process the bone pieces and interbody spaces, and the effects are not satisfying. It will be more difficult when handling the bony structures with the surgical instruments because they are sophisticated and expensive, and easy to be damaged. However, the spinal surgical instruments with conventional diameter can be applied and operated more flexibly in the working channel of the VBE system, which improves surgical efficiency, makes the interbody space treatment and the bony structure resection more satisfying and convenient, reduces the probability of surgical instrument damage, and eventually, expands the surgical indications and reduces the surgical cost.

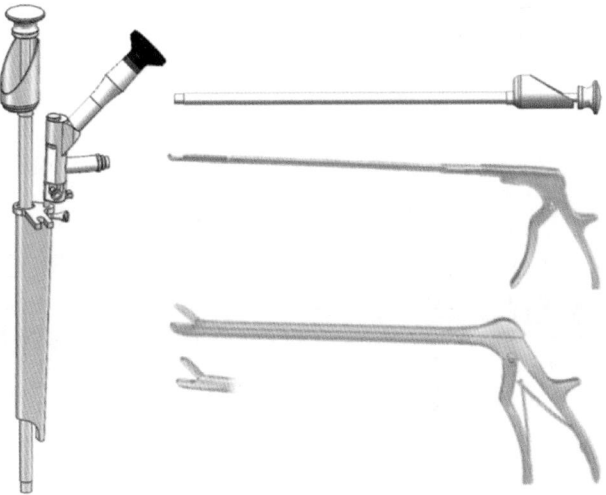

FIG. 2.13 Schematic diagram of conventional VBE surgical instruments.

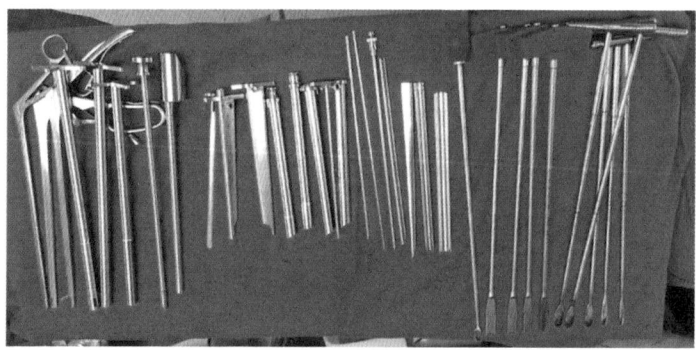

FIG. 2.14 Picture of conventional VBE surgical instruments.

2.2.5 The Water Plugs

A matching water plug is specially designed for the working channels of the bichannel endoscopy system, which can adjust the inner diameter of the working channel and water circulation simultaneously. The working channels can be adjusted to the desired size and position by inserting water plugs with different thicknesses or different shapes into the working channel (Figure 2.15). There are three types of water plugs. The first type is a large hollow water plug, which is mostly used for adjusting water circulation, blocking the dorsal part of the working channel at the front end to make it a closed space, and thus make the surgical field clearer. Additionally, conventional surgical instruments can be used in this situation because the central space of the large hollow water plug is large enough. The second type is a central hole water plug, which is mainly used for reducing the diameter of the working channel and decreasing the space of water circulation, which also makes the surgical view much clearer. The third type is an eccentric hole water plug. It not only reduces the diameter of the working channel or decreases the space of water circulation, but also allows the drills and other surgical instruments to be operated close to the edge of working channels, thus making the operation more flexible.

2.2.6 The Choice of Interbody Fusion Cages

The interbody implant includes the expandable and standard rigid interbody fusion cages. The expandable cages are the most used in clinical settings due to the limited size of the working channel. Currently, the expandable fusion cage can be made of different materials, including titanium ally, metal and PEEK materials, and some new types of expandable cage remain in the developing stages. During the operation, we just need to insert an expandable fusion cage with a height of 9–10 mm, and then expand it by 3–5 mm. Finally, the height of the expandable fusion cage can reach 12–14 mm, which can meet the needs of most patients with interbody fusion surgery (Figure 2.16). The original size of the standard rigid interbody fusion cage is relatively large, and it is difficult to implant a cage with a height of 12–14 mm during the operation. A larger diameter channel or special tools are required. This type of fusion cage is still used in clinics, but the dural sac needs to be properly retracted during the operation. If it is not operated under real-time endoscopic monitoring, the risk of neural injury is relatively high.

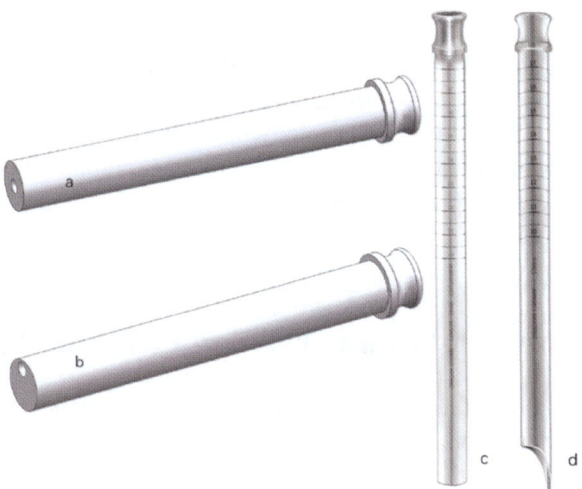

FIG. 2.15 Various matching water plugs for VBE.

(a) the central hole water plug; (b) the eccentric hole water plug; (c), (d) two types of large hollow water plug.

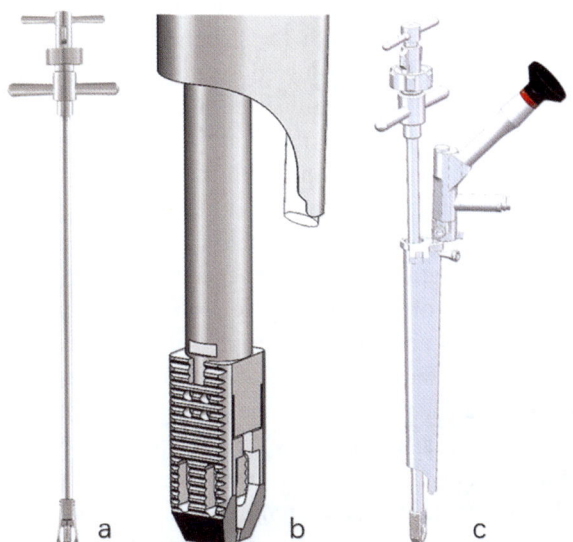

FIG. 2.16 The expandable fusion cage for VBE system.

(a) cage holder; (b), (c) insertion of the cage *via* VBE system.

2.2.7 Bone Graft Materials and Biological Factors

Two requirements should be met to achieve satisfactory interbody fusion, namely, excellent treatment of the interbody space and endplate, and sufficient bone graft materials (autogenous bone) are particularly preferred. When there is not enough autogenous bone to fill in the interbody space, allogeneic bone or artificial bone can be used. Moreover, factors that promote bone formation, such as bone morphogenetic protein (BMP) can also be used, if necessary. With the development of 3D printed fusion cages, there is no need for bone grafting, because the new bone can grow through the micropores. For endoscopy fusion, the autologous bone material may not be sufficient, because the bone obtained under minimally invasive conditions may be insufficient. At the moment, sufficient allogeneic bone should be supplemented, and bone formation factors such as BMP can also be added to further promote the interbody fusion.

2.3 Foraminoplasty and Working Cannula Placement

The key to the success of percutaneous endoscopic transforaminal discectomy (PETD) is to accurately place the working cannulas on the herniated nucleus pulposus. Kambin's triangle is a safe space that the working cannulas must pass through before approaching the lesion. It was first introduced by Dr. Parviz Kambin, and Kambin's triangle was defined as a right triangle over the dorsolateral disc [11]. The hypotenuse is the exiting nerve root, the base (width) is the superior border of the caudal vertebra and the height is the dura/traversing nerve root. The safer zone for placing the endoscope cannulas is in the medial aspect of Kambin's triangle, so the dimensions of the safe zone of the intervertebral foramina are very important for selecting a surgical instrument with an appropriate diameter. Mirkovic *et al.* conducted a study to investigate the intervertebral foraminal anatomy of L2-S1 and to determine the dimensions of the safe zone and the largest safe working cannula diameter of insertion [9]. The findings suggested that a 7.5 mm working cannula can be placed in line with the medial one third of the pedicle. Wimmer *et al.* found that the maximum safe working canula diameter is 8 mm for L1–L4, and 7 mm for L4-S1 by anatomic dissection [10]. Considering that the lower lumbar spine is more prone to degeneration than the upper lumbar spine, it is usually necessary to select a smaller diameter working cannula for the lower lumbar spine. Therefore, the hyperplasia of facet joints and the hypertrophy of the ligamentum flavum due to degeneration will further limit the size of the safe working zone. The upper part of the intervertebral foramina is mainly occupied by the exiting nerve roots, and the lower part of the intervertebral foramina is where the working cannula passes through. Since the intervertebral foramina window is narrow and the puncture path space is limited, only the slightly migrated disc herniation can be removed. In addition, for highly upward- or downward-migrated disc herniation, the difficulty is the establishment of an appropriate working channel, which might be impeded by normal anatomic structures at some times. This problematic issue can be solved by enlarging the foramen through foraminoplasty. For the uniportal and unichannel spinal endoscopy system, the bone drill is safer for the foraminoplasty, but is limited for the enlargement and formation of intervertebral foramen; while the trephine enables a greater degree of formation for the articular process, it increases the risk of neural injury under blind vision and X-ray radiation exposure to surgeons and patients by repeated fluoroscopy.

Kambin's triangle is considered a safe surgical space without important vascular and neural structures. This triangle can be used for epidural puncture of the poserolateral percutaneous foraminal approach, diagnostic imaging techniques, discectomy, and endoscopic lumbar interbody fusion. Since the 30° endoscopy system enters the intervertebral foramen, it always requires resection of a part of the facet joint to achieve proper visualization of the traversing nerve root. Kambin's original description of the triangle space neglected the fourth border of "the superior and inferior articular processes", so Kambin's triangle was essentially a two-dimensional triangular structure. When Andrew et al. added "the superior and inferior articular processes", Kambin's triangle became a truly three-dimensional structure and thus was named as "Kambin's Prism" [10]. The concept of Kambin's Prism has important anatomical significance for endoscopic lumbar interbody fusion. Fanous et al. proposed a new classification method according to the newly defined Kambin's Prism and the degree of the removal articular process [11]. Type I access (Kambin's Prism) has three approaches (Ia, Ib, and Ic). In type Ia access, the surgical corridor is parallel to the disc space. This is the approach used in percutaneous puncture, discogram, endoscopic discectomy, and intradiscal electrothermal therapy (IDET). In the second surgical approach that uses type I Kambin's Prism, type Ib access, the sagittal corridor is directed caudally. This approach is used to perform transforaminal microdiscectomy and transforaminal epidural steroid injections. It is the most common and most standard of all approaches that use Kambin's Prism to access spinal pathology. The third surgical approach that uses type I Kambin's Prism, type Ic access, is similar to type Ib access in that it is directed caudally in the sagittal plane, and the trajectory is more horizontal and aims for the spinal canal. This approach is used to perform endoscopic foraminotomy and endoscopic resection of the superior and inferior articular processes. In type II access, Kambin's Prism is expanded by removal of a limited amount of the lateral aspect of the inferior articular process of cephalad segment, and the lateral and anterior aspect of the superior articular process of the caudal segment. Type III access consists of the space obtained following complete removal of the superior and inferior articular processes along with the pars interarticularis and hemilamina. In the above classifications, type Ic access and type II access are mainly used for endoscopic lumbar interbody fusion.

2.4 Comparison of V-Shape Bichannel Endoscopy System and Conventional Unichannel Spinal Endoscopy Techniques

The uniportal and unichannel coaxial spinal endoscopy system is characterized by its minimal invasiveness and small surgical trauma. However, because of the above characteristics, the uniportal and unichannel spinal endoscopy sacrifices the surgical flexibility and efficiency. At the same time, the surgical instruments used are more sophisticated, which results in an increase in cost and the probability of surgical instrument damage. In contrast, the VBE system can increase the operational flexibility of endoscopic surgery and enables conventional instruments to be used, which will reduce the cost and the probability of surgical instrument damage. However, the surgical incision of the VBE technique is slightly more invasive than that of the uniaxial spinal endoscopy.

The VBE system is an enhancement and development of the coaxial spinal endoscopy system, which expands surgical indications. Specifically, for some simple spine surgeries, such as intervertebral disc removal and lateral spinal stenosis, the uniportal and unichannel coaxial spinal endoscopy system can fully meet the requirements and can achieve good clinical efficiency with minimal surgical incision. But for some complex spine surgeries and procedures, such as intervertebral fusion, the VBE system will work better than the uniportal and unichannel coaxial spinal endoscopy system. In addition, the VBE system is compatible with the existing uniportal and unichannel coaxial spinal endoscopy system, and all instruments and equipment of the uniportal and unichannel coaxial spinal endoscopy system can be used in the VBE system.

2.5 Comparison of V-Shape Bichannel Endoscopic Fusion and Unichannel Spinal Endoscopic Fusion

Conventional unichannel endoscopy-assisted lumbar fusion surgery reflects the minimally invasive advantages of fusion surgery. In 2016, Wang *et al.* conducted a study of 10 consecutive patients who received endoscopic foraminal decompression, lumbar interbody fusion, and percutaneous pedicle screw fixation with one year follow-up [12]. They demonstrated that with the use of this technique, the average hospital stay was reduced by over two days, and the postoperative recovery was also improved. However, when the research team completed 100 cases of patients treated with endoscopic fusion, they found two cases of interbody fusion cage migration, one case of endplate fracture, and one case of osteomyelitis during the follow-up period. Finally, they indicated that it was inefficient and time-consuming to perform procedures such as articular process resection, endplate preparation, and bone grafting, since the endoscopy diameter and the surgical instruments were small.

Currently, it has become mainstream for the unichannel endoscopic fusion to increase the diameter of the endoscope working channel to make it a wide-channel coaxial endoscope, and to become compatible with larger diameter surgical instruments based on the conventional uniportal and unichannel coaxial endoscopy. However, limited by the diameter of the endoscopy working channel, it is difficult to place the instruments with the same diameter as the conventional open surgery, including endplate reamer and fusion cage trial, through the endoscope channel from the tail end. Moreover, it is also difficult to directly place a fusion cage through the endoscope channel. Consequently, to complete the above procedures, the endoscope should be withdrawn and replaced by a larger working channel. It requires the surgeon's experience and repeated fluoroscopy to perform these operations under blind vision, which leads to an increased risk of neural injury and radiation exposure to surgeons and patients.

In comparison, the VBE system has an independent endoscopy channel and a working channel, which can be separated from each other. There is no need to customize the endoscopy due to changes in the diameter of the working channel, and just need to widen the diameter of working channel in the upper part of the cannula to place the instruments with the same diameter as the conventional open surgery. Moreover, the VBE system allows the surgical procedures, such as endplate preparation, placement of trial models, interbody bone grafting, implant of fusion cage, to be completed under full-time and real-time visualization. It is much more efficient and safer, and can significantly decrease the fluoroscopy frequency. Therefore, it can be really called "endoscopic" fusion instead of "endoscope-assisted" fusion.

2.6 Comparison of V-Shape Bichannel Endoscopy System and Unilateral Biportal Endoscopy Techniques

Unilateral biportal endoscopy (UBE) belongs to the unilateral independent biportal endoscopy technology of the posterior lumbar spine. Based on the anatomy of the posterior lumbar spine, two completely independent channels, namely an endoscopic channel and a working channel, are employed on the symptom side to visualize surgical procedures like the arthroscopic surgery (two-hole technology). The VBE technique is the inheritance and expansion of percutaneous endoscopic lumbar discectomy technology (uniportal and bichannel technology). For the UBE technique, the operating instrument is not limited by the size, and it can also be used for other procedures, such as endoscopic decompression and fusion. However, placing two channels during UBE procedures requires a learning curve combined with rich experience, both in arthroscopic technology and spine surgery technology. Essentially, the UBE technology needs a posterior interlaminar approach, and it requires a certain learning curve for some spine surgeons. By comparison, the VBE intervertebral foraminal path puncture technique will not increase the difficulty of puncture for most minimally invasive spine surgeons [13, 14].

Eum et al. believed that the UBE technique was more like a spinal microscope technique for surgeons [14]. It could achieve bilateral decompression through a unilateral approach, and has a smaller surgical incision, compared to the simple large channel decompression technique. Choi et al. conducted a prospective study to compare the levels of creatine phosphokinase (CPK) and C-reactive protein (CRP) in patients with lumbar disc herniation who underwent four surgical techniques, including microdiscectomy (MD), percutaneous endoscopic lumbar discectomy (PELD), percutaneous endoscopic interlaminar discectomy (PEID), and the UBE technique. The results suggested that PELD was the least invasive spinal surgical technique. Therefore, it can be shown that the VBE technique, which is directly inherited as a lateral transforaminal approach endoscopic technique, will be advantageous in invasive spine surgery [15].

In terms of microscopic fusion and surgical indications, the UBE technique is closer to the PLIF fusion, and has advantages in the treatment of central spinal stenosis. In contrast, the VBE technique is closer to the TLIF fusion, and has advantages in the treatment of lateral spinal stenosis and other cases that do not require extensive opening of the spine canal for decompression, such as lumbar spine instability and lumbar spondylolisthesis. Furthermore, the VBE technique, theoretically, can reduce immediate postoperative pain due to the stimulation of dural sac by bleeding, and the long-term intractable low back pain caused by the dural sac and nerve root adhesion after lumbar spine surgery.

In summary, the V-shape bichannel endoscopy system (VBE) has the following functions as compared with the existing spinal endoscopy system. First, it expands the surgical indications of spinal endoscopy, especially for application in complex spinal surgeries. Second, it enables the application of surgical instruments with conventional diameter, thus reducing the probability and the cost of surgical instrument damage. Third, it increases the safety and efficiency of the surgical procedures with conventional surgical instruments used under the full-time and real-time monitoring of the endoscope.

References

[1] Forst R., Hausmann B. (1983) Nucleoscopy–A new examination technique, *Arch Orthop Trauma Surg.* **101**(3), 219.

[2] De Antoni D.J., Claro M.L., Poehling G.G., *et al.* (1996) Translaminar lumbar epidural endoscopy: Anatomy, technique, and indications, *Arthroscopy* **12**(3), 330.

[3] Yeung A.T. (1999) Minimally invasive disc surgery with the yeung endoscopic spine system (YESS), *Surg. Technol. Int.* **8**, 267.

[4] Kim M.J., Lee S.H., Jung E.S., *et al.* (2007) Targeted percutaneous transforaminal endoscopic diskectomy in 295 patients: Comparison with results of microscopic discectomy, *Surg. Neurol.* **68**(6), 623.

[5] Osman S.G. (2012) Endoscopic transforaminal decompression, interbody fusion, and percutaneous pedicle screw implantation of the lumbar spine: A case series report, *Int. J. Spine Surg.* **6**, 157.

[6] Kitahama Y., Sairyo K., Dezawa A. (2013) Percutaneous endoscopic transforaminal approach to decompress the lateral recess in an elderly patient with spinal canal stenosis, herniated nucleus pulposus and pulmonary comorbidities, *Asian J. Endosc. Surg.* **6**(2), 130.

[7] Ahn Y. (2014) Percutaneous endoscopic decompression for lumbar spinal stenosis, *Expert Rev. Med. Devices* **11**(6), 605.

[8] Lewandrowski K.U. (2014) "Outside-in" technique, clinical results, and indications with transforaminal lumbar endoscopic surgery: A retrospective study on 220 patients on applied radiographic classification of foraminal spinal stenosis. *Int. J. Spine Surg.* **8**.

[9] Mirkovic S.R., Schwartz D.G., Glazier K.D. (1995) Anatomic considerations in lumbar posterolateral percutaneous procedures, *Spine (Phila Pa 1976)*, **20**(18), 1965.

[10] Wimmer C., Maurer H. (2000) Anatomic consideration for lumbar percutaneous interbody fusion, *Clin. OrthopRelat. Res.* (379) 236.

[11] Fanous A.A., Tumialan L.M., Wang M.Y. (2019) Kambin's triangle: Definition and new classification schema. *J. Neurosurg. Spine* 1.

[12] Wang M.Y., Grossman J. (2016) Endoscopic minimally invasive transforaminal interbody fusion without general anesthesia: Initial clinical experience with 1-year follow-up, *Neurosurg. Focus* **40**(2), E13.

[13] Kolcun J.P.G., Brusko G.D., Basil G.W., *et al.* (2019) Endoscopic transforaminal lumbar interbody fusion without general anesthesia: Operative and clinical outcomes in 100 consecutive patients with a minimum 1-year follow-up, *Neurosurg. Focus* **46**, E14.

[14] Hwa Eum J., Hwa Heo D., Son S.K., *et al.* (2016) Percutaneous biportal endoscopic decompression for lumbar spinal stenosis: A technical note and preliminary clinical results, *J. Neurosurg. Spine* **24**(4), 602.

[15] Choi K.C., Shim H.K., Hwang J.S., Shin S.H., Lee D.C., Jung H.H., Park H.A., Park C.K. (2018) Comparison of surgical invasiveness between microdiscectomy and 3 different endoscopic discectomy techniques for lumbar disc herniation, *World Neurosurg.* **116**, e750.

Chapter 3

Clinical Applied Anatomy for V-Shape Bichannel Endoscopy

Section Editors:

Qun Yang, MD
Haijian Ni, MD
Bo Wang, MD
Yunshan Fan, MD

3.1 General Anatomy of the Lumbosacral Spine

The lumbosacral including the lumbar and sacral spine, is the lowest part of the spine. It has both weight-bearing and motion functions. Normally, the lumbar section contains five lumbar vertebrae. Each lumbar vertebra consists of a vertebral body and some appendages at the posterior side of the vertebral body. The pedicle, lamina, and the posterior margin of the vertebral body form the vertebral foramen. Adjacent vertebral foramina form the spinal canal, which accommodates the spinal cord and nerves. There are discs lying between adjacent lumbar vertebrae and between the fifth lumbar (L5) and the first sacral (S1) vertebra. The sacrum is comprised of five vertebrae that fuse during adulthood. Except the lumbosacral joint between S1 and L5, the sacrum also forms the left and right sacroiliac joints with the ilium, through which the gravity of the trunk can be transferred to the lower extremities. The sacrum is also connected to the coccyx by joint and ligaments.

3.1.1 Bone Structures of the Lumbosacral Spine

(1) The vertebral body

The lumbar vertebrae bodies are the largest in the spine. The sagittal and transverse diameters of the lower vertebra are greater than those of the upper vertebra. The transverse diameter of a vertebral body is larger than its' sagittal diameter. The lumbar vertebral bodies are in elliptic or renal shape in the cross section. The anterior vertebral body height increases, while the posterior vertebral body height decreases from the first to the fifth lumbar vertebra, and that forms the lumbar lordosis.

(2) The vertebral pedicle

The vertebral pedicle protrudes from the posterolateral side of the vertebral body. Each vertebral pedicle has two notches, the superior and inferior notches, which form the lower and the upper borders of the intervertebral foramen, respectively. The superior notch is smaller than the inferior notch. The sagittal diameter of the superior notch gradually decreases from the first lumbar vertebra, while that of the inferior notch of adjacent vertebrae has no significant difference. The width of the lateral recess can be estimated from the sagittal diameter of the corresponding superior notch.

(3) The lamina

The lamina of the lumbar vertebra is thick and slopes slightly backward. Normally, the thickness of a lamina is no more than 8 mm. The angle between the left and right laminae is about 83°–90°. A smaller angle may cause spinal stenosis.

(4) Facet joint (zygapophysial joint)

The superior facet emanates from the vertebral pedicle. The inferior facet originates from the junction of the vertebral pedicle and the lamina. The superior and inferior articular processes are interconnected by pars interarticularis. The superior and inferior facets mostly lie in the sagittal plane, and gradually become oblique from L1 to L5, almost in the coronal plane at L5. Spinal stenosis can result from the hyperosteogeny of the superior facet or the forward slip of the inferior facet.

(5) The transverse process

The transverse process protrudes outward from the junction of the pedicle and the lamina, except the transverse process of the fifth vertebra, which originates from the junction of the pedicle and the vertebral body. The transverse process of the third vertebra is the longest. The oval bulge on the posterior margin of the superior articular process is the mamillary process. The small tubercle on the posteroinferior side of the transverse process is the accessory process.

(6) The spinous process

The spinous process of the lumbar vertebra is relatively short. It is in the horizontal plane, and slightly slopes downward. With ligaments and muscles attached to it, the spinous process plays an important role in maintaining the stability of the posterior structure of spine. In patients with thin subcutaneous fat, the palpation of the spinous process can be used for the preoperative lumbar spine level localization.

(7) The spinal canal

The vertebral body and its posterior appendages form the vertebral foramen. Connected vertebral foramina form the spinal canal, which accommodates the spinal cord and nerves. The spinal canal can be divided into central canal and lateral canal. The central canal is occupied by the spinal cord with the dural sac surrounded. The lateral canal is the lateral part of the spinal nerve root canal. The lateral canal is also known as lateral recess in the lower lumbar spine. The anterior border of the lateral recess is the posterior aspect of the vertebral body. The posterior border of the lateral recess is the junction of the anteroinferior aspect of the superior articular facet, the pedicle, and the lamina. The lateral side of the lateral recess is the medial side of the pedicle, and the medial entrance of the lateral recess corresponds to the anterior edge of the superior articular process (Figure 3.1). Nerve compression secondary to lateral recess stenosis is one of the causes of low back pain and lower extremities pain.

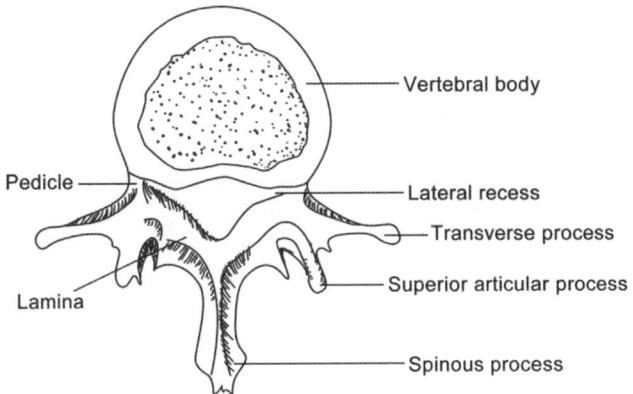

FIG. 3.1 Structure of the lumbosacral vertebra.

3.1.2 Connections Between Vertebrae

(1) The intervertebral disc

The intervertebral disc is a structure connecting two adjacent vertebrae. The intervertebral disc consists of cartilage plates, annulus fibrosus, and nucleus pulposus. Physiologically, the intervertebral disc is elastic. It can relieve and absorb the shock of external forces on the spine and the spinal cord while participating in the motor function of the spine (Figure 3.2). Degeneration and injuries of the intervertebral disc are considered as the initiating factors of degenerative spinal diseases.

1) The cartilaginous plate, also known as the endplate, is the cartilaginous surface of hyaline cartilage covering the upper and lower surfaces of the vertebral body. The cartilaginous plate acts as a semi-permeable membrane through which water and nutrients can penetrate the inner layer of the nucleus pulposus and the annulus fibrosus, which have no direct blood supply. When the endplate is torn, the nucleus pulposus may herniate into the vertebral body and form the Schmorl-nodule.

2) The annulus fibrosus is fibrous tissue arranged in concentric circles, closely connected with the upper and lower cartilaginous plates and the anterior and posterior longitudinal ligaments. The annulus fibrosus has anti-rotation and anti-twist features. Each layer of the annulus fibrosus crisscrosses each other diagonally (about 30°). The innermost fibers fuse with the intercellular matrix of the nucleus pulposus without an obvious boundary. Physiologically, there are no blood vessels or nerve endings in the inner third of the annulus fibrosus. However, tears of the inner annulus fibrosus due to

trauma, degeneration or other factors, may lead to proliferation of blood vessels and nerve endings, which is the pathological basis of the discogenic pain.

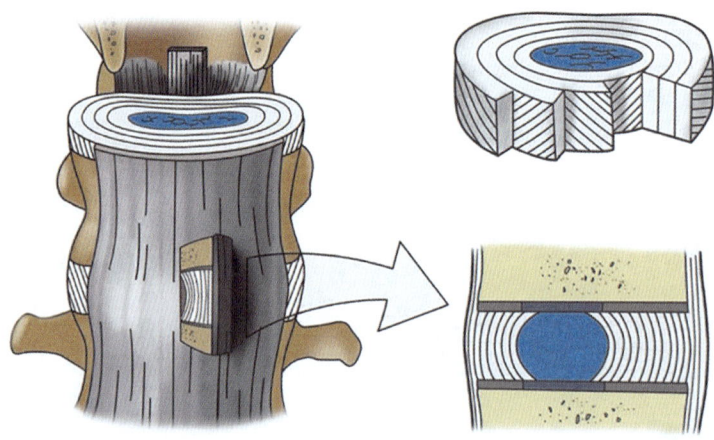

FIG. 3.2   The structure of the lumbar intervertebral disc.

3) The nucleus pulposus is formed of elastic jelly substance, consisting of water (85%) and other elements such as chondrocytes, proteoglycans, and chondroitin sulfate. The water content of the nucleus pulposus decreases with age, and so does the elasticity of the disc. Therefore, disruption of the annulus fibrosus, and herniation or protrusion of the nucleus pulposus, which can lead to symptoms of nerve compression, are more likely to occur due to trauma or degenerative factors.

(2) The ligament

1) The anterior longitudinal ligament runs down the ventral side of the spine. It is strong and the longest ligament in the human body. It can be divided into three layers: the superficial fibers spanning three to five vertebral bodies, the intermediate fibers spanning two to three vertebral bodies, and the intersegmental deep fibers spanning one intervertebral disc. The anterior longitudinal ligament holds the vertebrae and intervertebral discs tightly together and limits the hyperextension of the spine.

2) The posterior longitudinal ligament is located posterior to the vertebral bodies with uneven width. The posterior longitudinal ligament cannot completely cover the posterior part of the vertebral bodies and intervertebral discs. The superficial fibers of the posterior longitudinal ligament can span three to four vertebral bodies. The dentate deep fibers connect to adjacent vertebrae and often have cracks, allowing the basivertebral veins to pass through. The posterior longitudinal ligament mainly limits the hyperflexion of the spine.

3) The supraspinous ligament and the interspinous ligament connect the apex of the spinous processes and the spinous processes, respectively. The interspinous ligament

transits to the ligamentum flavum anteriorly and to the supraspinous ligament posteriorly. The supraspinous ligament and the interspinous ligament can limit the hyperflexion of the spine.

4) The intertransverse process ligament connects transverse processes of adjacent vertebrae. It can be divided into the medial part and the lateral part. The medial part has tendinous arches protecting the posterior branches of spinal nerves and blood vessels. The intertransverse process ligament is a dysplastic thin fascia layer at the lateral clearance of the lumbar transverse process. The intertransverse process ligament participates in the formation of the iliolumbar ligament between the transverse processes of L4 and L5, and forms the lumbosacral portion of the iliolumbar ligament between L5 and S1.

5) The ligamentum flavum is composed of yellow elastic fiber tissues located between the laminae of adjacent vertebrae. The ligamentum flavum is flat in shape, and thickened from L1 to S1. The ligamentum flavum attaches to the anteroinferior surface of the cephalad lamina, extends outward to the root of the inferior articular process and the root of the transverse process of the same cephalad vertebra, and inserts into the posterosuperior surface of the caudal lamina and the anterosuperior capsule of the superior articular process. The ligamentum flavum forms the posterior and posterolateral walls of the spinal canal, maintains the normal alignment of the vertebrae, and limits the hyperflexion of the spine. Due to degeneration or external factors, the ligamentum flavum may become thickened and less elastic, leading to spinal stenosis and nerve compression.

(3) The facet joints

The facet joint, or the zygapophyseal joint, is formed by adjacent superior and inferior articular facets of two vertebrae. A facet joint includes two articular surfaces, a joint capsule, and some synovial tissues. The lumbar facet joint is usually oriented in the oblique sagittal plane, which allows the facet joint to flex, extend, and flex laterally. However, in the lower lumbar region, especially in L5/S1 or in sacralization of the lumbar vertebra, the facet joint can be almost in the coronal plane. This may be related to the degeneration of corresponding segments.

3.1.3 The Spinal Cord and Nerves of the Lumbosacral Spine

(1) The spinal cord

There is an enlargement called the intumescentia lumbalis at the lower part of the spinal cord, usually at the level of T10 to L1. The intumescentia lumbalis gradually becomes conical at the lumbar segment and forms the conus medullaris. In adults, the conus medullaris is generally located approximately at the level of L1. The filum terminale, a filament of connective tissue, extends from the apex of the conus medullaris. After originating from the spinal cord, the lumbar, sacral, and caudal nerve roots travel a long distance around the filum finalis along the spinal canal and exit through the corresponding intervertebral foramina. The bundle of nerve roots in the spinal canal is called the cauda equina.

(2) The spinal nerve

The spinal nerve root is composed of the ventral root and the dorsal root, wrapped by the spinal pia mater, arachnoid, and the spinal dura mater. The nerve fibers of the ventral root come from the anterior horn of the spinal cord. Ventral roots mainly innervate the peripheral muscles and control the motor function. The dorsal root mainly contains sensory afferent fibers with their primary neurons located at the dorsal root ganglion. The dorsal roots enter the spinal cord at the posterolateral sulcus. The ventral root and the dorsal root confluence and form the spinal nerve, which exits from the corresponding intervertebral foramen. The following are main branches of the spinal nerve.

1) The ventral ramus, or the anterior branch, mainly innervates the muscles of the trunk and lower extremities, and participates in the composition of the lumbosacral plexus.

2) The dorsal ramus, or the posterior branch, contains sensory fibers with endings distribute in the joint capsule, skin, and other receptors. It can be further divided into the medial branch and the lateral branch.

3) The rami communicans, or the communicating branches, are fine branches between the spinal nerve and the sympathetic trunk. The branches connecting the spinal nerve to the sympathetic trunk are the white rami communicans. The branches connecting the sympathetic trunk to the spinal nerve are the gray rami communicans.

4) The meningeal branch, also called the recurrent branch, is a branch that reenters the intervertebral foramen after it originates from the spinal nerve. It serves the synovium, ligaments, and other tissues in the spinal canal. The meningeal branch containing sensory fibers from the spinal nerve, as well as fibers connecting the adjacent sympathetic ganglion, is called the sinuvertebral nerve (Figure 3.3). The sinuvertebral nerve innervates the meninges, the posterior longitudinal ligament, the intervertebral disc, blood vessels and other tissues. It may lead to back pain when the sinuvertebral nerve is stimulated because of intervertebral disc disorder.

3.1.4 *The Vascular Distribution in the Lumbosacral Spine*

(1) Segmental vessels

The lumbar segmal arteries emanate from the aorta abdominalis, and are arranged symmetrically along both sides of the vertebral body. The lumbar segmal arteries mainly supply the lumbar spine, paravertebral muscles, and retroperitoneal muscles. The lumbar segmal arteries have accompanying veins; however, the segmental veins are rarely in pairs, because of the high proportion of variations and the relatively unstable positions. The segmental veins are more likely to appear on the left side than on the right; therefore, blood flowing into the inferior vena cava is more likely through the left segmental veins.

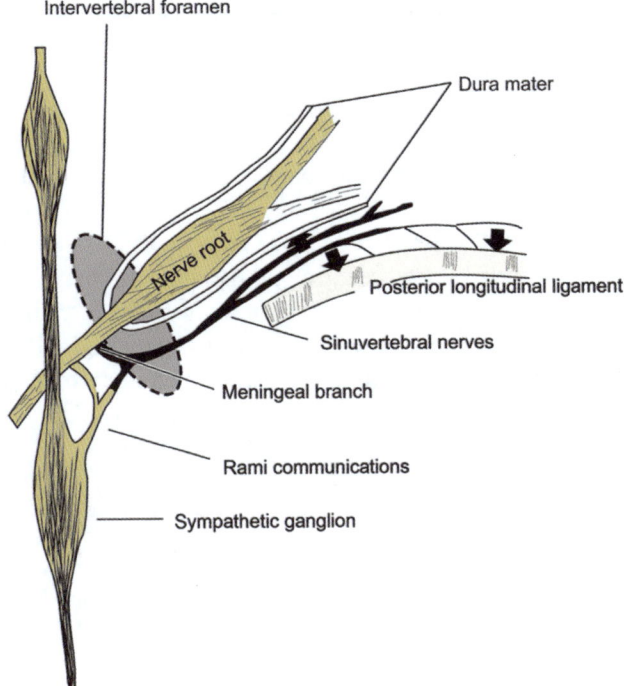

FIG. 3.3 The sinuvertebral nerve.

(2) Branches of the segmental vessels

The segmental arteries are generally distributed in pairs. The trunk of the segmental artery originates from the aorta abdominalis and then goes backward along the center of the vertebral body. Near the anterolateral margin of the intervertebral foramen, the trunk of the segmental artery gives off three main branches: the anterior transverse process branch, the dorsal branch, and the spinal branch (Figure 3.4). The anterior transverse process branch is relatively large and lies along the anterior edge of transverse process. The dorsal branch travels backward, bypasses the isthmus of the lamina, and supplies the superior and inferior articular processes. The dorsal branch also gives off branches supplying the posterior muscles, ligaments, and soft tissues. The spinal branch enters the intervertebral foramen and gives off three branches. One goes ventrally to supply the posterior of the vertebral body, one goes dorsally to supply the lamina and the ligamentum flavum, and the rest one goes in parallel with the spinal nerve root to the proximal end of the nerve root. The nerve root is not only supplied by arterial branches from the distal and lateral side, but also by branches of the anterior and posterior spinal arteries from the proximal side. The proximal and distal branches form the arterial system supplying the nerve root together.

The venous system of the lumbosacral vertebra consists of the external vertebral venous plexus and the internal vertebral venous plexus. The external vertebral venous plexus surrounds the lateral side of the vertebral body and mainly flows into the ascending lumbar veins. The external vertebral venous plexus can be divided into the anterior and the posterior external vertebral plexuses according to their positional relationships with the vertebral body. The anterior and posterior external vertebral plexuses communicate with the segmental veins and the internal vertebral venous plexus through the foramen and other bony and fiber channels. The internal vertebral venous plexus is located on the medial side of the bony structure of the intervertebral foramen and is surrounded by a small collection of loose adipose tissues. The internal vertebral venous plexus can be divided into three groups: the anterior internal vertebral venous plexus, the posterior internal vertebral venous plexus, and the spinal radicular veins (Figure 3.5). The radicular veins are segmental veins, which go along the upper and lower sides of the pedicles of the vertebral arch and penetrate through the intervertebral foramen. The internal vertebral venous plexus is characterized by the absence of venous valves.

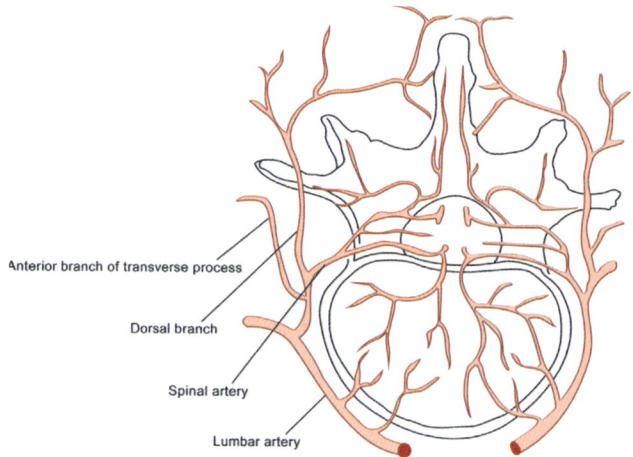

FIG. 3.4   Arteries of the lumbosacral vertebra.

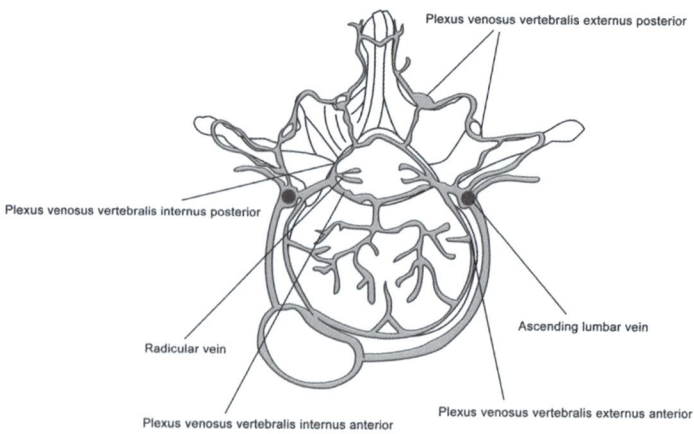

FIG. 3.5   Veins of the lumbosacral vertebra.

3.2 Anatomy Related to V-Shape Bichannel Endoscopy Surgical Approaches

The first coaxial spinal endoscopic system (Yeung Endoscopic Spine System, YESS) was developed in the mid and late 1990s. YESS allows surgeons to puncture and catheterize into the intervertebral disc under the guidance of fluoroscopy. Hoogland invented Thomas Hoogland Endoscopy Spine System (THESYS) in 2002. THESYS places the channel more dorsolateral, to make the channel reach the spinal canal directly through the intervertebral foramen and direct decompression can be performed. This is called the TESSYS technique. Partial resection of the articular process is often required to enlarge the intervertebral foramen for the catheterization due to view obstruction of the articular process on the dorsal side. The core of the TESSYS technique is to perform decompression directly in the spinal canal by removing part of the articular process and placing the channel more dorsally. This technique expands the indications for the transforaminal endoscopic surgery.

However, the TESSYS technique still has some inadequacies. First of all, repeated X-ray fluoroscopy is required in the process of the catheterization, which brings a relatively large amount of radiation exposure to both patients and surgeons. Secondly, foraminoplasty (resection of the articular process) was not very efficient. The slope of the lateral facet makes it easy to slide to the ventral side during foraminoplasty. Furthermore, the whole procedure of the resection is performed non-visually under X-ray fluoroscopy whether it is using a trephine or a drill. This drawback increases the risk of nerve injury. It is difficult to become proficient with TESSYS technique in a short time due to these inadequacies. The learning curve of the TESSYS technique is steep.

To solve the above inadequacies, the VBE system came into being. Following the conventional surgical principle of entering from the outside to the inside layer by layer, the VBE system can reach the surgical site with neither the precise puncture under repeated fluoroscopy, nor the step-by-step non-visual resection of the articular process with a trephine or a drill. With the VBE system, simply by directing the working cannula to the anterolateral side of the superior articular process, the surgeon can perform the resection of the articular process and then enter the spinal canal under the full supervision through a secondary channel with observation endoscope. Therefore, the core advantages of the VBE system can be summarized as: more stable operation on the dorsal spine, more efficient resection of the articular process and follow-up operations, and safer full visualization [1, 2].

The approach of VBE surgeries, whether the endoscopic discectomy or fusion, involves the intervertebral foramen, articular process, safety triangle, and other related structures, anatomies of which are described as follows.

3.2.1 Anatomy of the Lumbar Intervertebral Foramen

The lumbar intervertebral foramen is a bony foramen formed by adjacent vertebrae at the lateral side of the lumbar spine. It is the channel through which spinal nerve roots pass obliquely after originating from the dural sac. The anatomy of the foraminal region is complex, which make iatrogenic injuries, such as nerve and vascular damage prone when surgical procedures are performed in this region. Therefore, the surgeon must be acquainted with the anatomy and possible variations of the foraminal region to perform a VBE surgery successfully and avoid related complications [3, 4].

(1) Gross morphology of the lumbar intervertebral foramen

Reports on the boundaries and morphology of the lumbar intervertebral foramen are not completely consistent in different literatures. Generally, the superior and inferior boundaries of the lumbar intervertebral foramen are enclosed by inferior notch of upper pedicle and superior notch of lower pedicle of two adjacent lumbar vertebrae. The anterior boundary is formed by the posterolateral side of the adjacent vertebral bodies, the dorsal part of the intervertebral disc, and the posterior longitudinal ligament. The posterior boundary is the capsule of the facet joint and the ligamentum flavum covers the front of the facet joint. The medial side of the intervertebral foramen is towards the spinal canal, and on the lateral side, there is a layer of connective tissue. The lumbar nerve root, sinuvertebral nerve, lumbar arteries, veins, lymphatics, and adipose tissues enter or exit the foramen through the lateral area.

The average height, width, and area of the lumbar intervertebral foramen of Chinese people are 13–16 mm, 7–9 mm, and 83–103 mm^2, respectively. The intervertebral foramen of L2/L3 is the largest, and both the height and width of the lumbar intervertebral forammen increase from L1/2 to L2/3, and gradually decrease from L2/L3 to L5/S1. Normally, lumbar intervertebral foramen is more elliptic than renal shaped; however, they become significantly more renal or auricular than elliptic shaped when the intervertebral disc and/or facet joint are abnormal. The area of the lumbar intervertebral foramen will gradually decrease with age and degeneration. Compared with the anteroposterior diameter, the suprainferior diameter decreases more significantly with age. The area of the lumbar intervertebral foramen can also change with flexion and extension of the spine mediated by two mobilizable structures, the disc, and the facet joint. In general, the area of the intervertebral foramen increases in the flexion state of the spine and decreases in the hyperextension state of the spine [5].

(2) Lumbar intervertebral foraminal ligaments

In 1969, Colub anatomically studied the lumbar intervertebral foramen and firstly discovered the ligamentous structures within the foramen [6]. At that time, however, Colub believed that these ligamentous structures were just pathological tissues, due to the lack of clear patterns in their distribution. With the development of research, the ligaments were normal anatomical structures of the intervertebral foramen. Foraminal ligaments exist on both sides of and also run through the lumbar intervertebral foramen. The foraminal ligaments have no muscle attachments, and the ligaments in the upper lumbar foramina are more rounded, thick, and clear than those in the lower lumbar foramina. Bounded by the vertical line passing through the medial edge of the upper and lower pedicle and the vertical line passing through the lateral edge of the upper and lower pedicle, the intervertebral foramen can be divided into three areas. These are the entrance area, the central area and the exit area. The foraminal ligaments are found in all three regions, and are called the internal foraminal, intraforaminal, and external foraminal ligaments, respectively [7-9].

1) The internal foraminal ligaments include the lateral extension of the posterior longitudinal ligaments in the front and the ligamentum flavum in the rear, as well as ligaments underneath the intervertebral foramen connecting the posterolateral side of the disc to the front of the superior articular process.The medial ligaments radially surround the nerve root and fix it in the intervertebral foramen in different directions with a certain tension, so as to stabilize and protect the nerve root.

2) The intraforaminal ligaments mainly include the radial ligaments and the extension of the ligamentum flavum to the foramen. The anterior intraforaminal ligament attaches from the root of the pedicle to the lower boundary of the same vertebral body. The pores formed by the ligaments and vertebrae are crossed by a branch of the spinal artery and the recurrent branch of the spinal nerve. The superior intraforaminal ligament, the posterior end of the pedicle, and the root of the transverse process form an anterosuperior compartment, through which a large branch of the segmental artery passes. There is another type of intraforaminal ligament originating from the anterior upper portion of the superior articular process and attaching on the posterolateral surface of the upper vertebral body, above which the spinal nerve penetrates through the foramen intervertebral.

3) The external foraminal ligaments include the superior and inferior transverse foramen ligaments. The superior transverse foramen ligament is located at the upper part of the external area of the intervertebral foramen. It crosses the inferior notch of the vertebral arch and attaches from the lateral edge of the isthmus to the superolateral surface of the vertebral body of the same segment, the annulus fibrosus of the disc, and the lateral side of the posterior longitudinal ligament. The inferior transverse foramen ligament sometimes consists of two ligaments, or two ligaments coalesce into a horizontal "Y" shape. The inferior transverse foramen ligament starts from the junction of the upper portion of the root of the transverse process and the superior articular process, and the anterior bone surface of the superior articular process, and attaches to the caudal vertebral body, the annulus fibrosus of the disc and the lateral side of the posterior longitudinal ligament. The ligaments above generally separate the external area of the intervertebral foramen into three compartments, among which the large central compartment has spinal nerves and the spinal branch of the segmental artery passing through, while the two smaller compartments, the superior and inferior compartments, have corresponding drainage veins passing through.

(3) Nerves of the lumbar intervertebral foramen

Spinal nerve roots usually go through the superior portion of the lumbar intervertebral foramen. Spinal nerve roots include the anterior motor root and the posterior sensory root connected to the anterolateral and posterolateral sulcus spinal cord, respectively. The nerve roots are anchored by Hoffmann's ligaments and can move with postural changes of the spine. In the sensory root, there is a dorsal root ganglion, the size of which gradually increases from the lower to the upper lumbar spine. At the foramen, the anterior motor root combines with the posterior sensory root distal to the dorsal root ganglion to form the mixed spinal nerve. The spinal nerve usually gives off the anterior rami and the posterior rami in the exit area of the foramen. The recurrent meningeal nerves branch from the spinal nerve before the origin site of the anterior and posterior rami. The meningeal branches go in the opposite direction with the nerve trunk. They return to the spinal canal through the intervertebral foramen, and innervate the spinal dura mater, the adventitia of spinal nerve roots, spinal vessels, and the vertebral periosteum. The recurrent meningeal branches of the spinal nerve contain abundant sensory and sympathetic fibers, which may cause pain of the low back or the lower extremities when stimulated.

(4) **Blood vessels of the lumbar intervertebral foramen**

The lumbar arteries usually travel close to the vertebral body. The first to fourth lumbar arteries emanate from the abdominal aorta, and the fifth lumbar artery emanates from the median sacral artery. The radicular artery arises from the spinal branch of the lumbar artery, usually accompanied by the spinal nerve root. After penetrating the intervertebral foramen into the spinal canal, the radicular artery gives off the anterior and posterior radicular arteries and the spinal meningeal branch. There are many veins in the foramen, which can be divided into two categories. One category is the communicating venous plexus, which is an important venous channel connecting the internal and external venous plexus of the spinal canal. The communicating venous plexus has no venous valve, and it mainly passes through the compartment formed by the internal ligaments and the superior notch of the pedicle. The other category is the radicular vein, which usually exits through the posteroinferior portion of the foramen with the nerve root.

3.2.2 Anatomy of the Lumbar Facet Joint

The paired facet joints of two consecutive lumbar vertebrae and the intervertebral disc between them form the lumbar three-joint complex. According to biomechanical studies, the lumbar three-joint complex plays an important role in maintaining the stability and motor function of the lumbar spine. The facet joints of the lumbar spine are true joints with a considerable range of motion (ROM). The lumbar facet joints and their appendages are the main structures forming the posterior wall of the foramen. Partial or complete resection of the articular facets is often required during VBE decompression or fusion; therefore, it is necessary to be familiar with the anatomy of the lumbar facet joint.

(1) **The articular facet**

The articular facets of two adjacent vertebrae are covered with articular cartilage and combined by concave-convex connection. The articular cartilage extends to the periphery of the articular surface in a crescent shape, and makes the rough osseous articular surface more closely aligned to reduce the friction, and therefore, conduce better joint movement and stability.

(2) **The capsule of the facet joint**

The anterior and posterior walls of lumbar facet joint capsule are tense, while the upper and lower walls are slack. The ligamentum flavum extends outward and integrates with the anterior wall. It also extends inward to the lamina, and outward to the front of the superior facet to strengthen the anterior wall. There is no significant difference in the thickness of the joint capsule in each segment. The multifidus muscles attach from the lateral sides of the superior and posterior walls of the joint capsule and to the spinous process of the vertebrae two or three levels above.

(3) The cavity of the facet joint

In the cross section, the space between the cartilage covering the superior and inferior articular facet is about 0.5 mm in height. The cavity is narrow in front, wide in back, and enlarges from the upper to the lower lumbar spine. From the coronal and sagittal plane, the superior and inferior poles of the joint cavity form a latent recess filled with synovial plica. The incarceration of the synovial plica may cause severe pain.

(4) The articular synovium

Like other joints, the articular synovium of the facet joint attaches to the periphery of the articular cartilage. A part of the synovium returns to the articular cavity and forms the synovial plica, the size of which varies with the degree of articular combination. The synovial plica of the superior and inferior poles of the joint cavity is broad and large, while the synovial plica of the anterior and posterior of the cavity is relatively small, and generally does not protrude into the articular cavity.

3.2.3 The Safety Triangle

Early researchers found complications of nerve injuries in patients who received intervertebral disc interventions, such as intervertebral disc injection, incision and aspiration, through the lateral approach. Based on anatomical studies of the surgical approach, Kambin firstly proposed the concept of the safety triangle, which was described as a triangular area surrounded by the superior surface of the lamina of the lower vertebra, the spinal dural sac/traversing nerve root, and the exiting nerve root. It is relatively safe to puncture in this triangular area. This safety triangle is called Kambin's triangle by later researchers. However, if the superior articular facet is considered, the dorsal side of Kambin's triangle is actually the ventral side of the superior articular process in the lateral view. The articular process will be an obstacle for endoscopic decompression or fusion through the transforaminal approach, which requires a larger working space. Partial or complete resection of the articular process is usually required. Some researchers proposed the concepts of the intervertebral foramen safety triangle and intraspinal safety triangle. The intervertebral foramen safety triangle is defined as the triangular area composed of the superior surface of the lamina of the lower vertebra as the base of the triangle, the facet joint as the height, and the exiting nerve root as the hypotenuse. The intraspinal safety triangle is defined as the triangular area composed of the superior surface of the lamina of the lower vertebra as the base, the spinal dural sac/ traversing nerve root as the medial side, and the exiting nerve root as the hypotenuse [10].

In VBE endoscopic fusion surgery, the risk of nerve injury mainly focuses on the exiting root. From L1 to S1, the exiting nerve root angle becomes narrower because the intervertebral foramen gets further away from the originating point of the corresponding nerve root. Therefore, the more caudal to the lumbar segment, the lower the channel to the ventral side, which can make the target operation area closer to the inner side, so as to obtain greater operation space. The exiting nerve roots of L1–L3 are relatively horizontal at the exit of the intervertebral foramen, because they originate from a lower position of the intervertebral space. Therefore, special attention should be paid to avoid injury to the exiting nerve root. In addition, due to the small width of the facet joint, the side opening distance of the endoscopic channel should not be too large, otherwise it may also lead to dural sac/traversing nerve root injury.

References

[1] Ye J., Lin P., Xie Q., et al. (2001) Anatomic orientation of lumbar facet joints and its effects on degeneration of intervertebral disc [in Chinese], *J. Fujian Medical Univ.* **35**(4), 326.

[2] Min J., Kang S., Lee J., et al. (2005) Morphometric analysis of the working zone for endoscopic lumbar discectomy, *J. Spinal Disord Tech.* **18**(2), 132.

[3] Yuan S., Li Y., Wang, et al. (2010) Applied anatomy of intrusive operations of lumbar intervertebral foramen [in Chinese], *Chin. J. Clin. Anat.* **28**(2), 127.

[4] Civelek E., Solmaz I., Cansever T., et al. (2012) Radiological analysis of the triangular working zone during transforaminal endoscopic lumbar discectomy, *Asian Spine J.* **6**(2), 98.

[5] Hardenbrook M., Lombardo S., Wilson M., et al. (2016) The anatomic rationale for transforaminal endoscopic interbody fusion: A cadaveric analysis, *Neurosurg. Focus* **E12**, 40.

[6] Golub B.S., Silverman B. (1969) Transforaminal ligaments of the lumbar spine, *J. Bone Joint Surg Am.* **51**(5), 947.

[7] Zhao Q., Lv H., Ding Z. (2018) Review in the clinical anatomy of the L5~S1 intervertebral foramen ligament [in Chinese], *Chin. Clin. Anat.* **36**(2), 231.

[8] Yin S., Li J., Zhang X. (2018) Anatomy and clinical significance of spinal intervertebral foramen ligament [in Chinese], *J. Inner Mongolia Medical Univ.* **40**(3), 313.

[9] Feng Y., Li H., Li Y. (2019) Applied anatomy of the lumbar intervertebral foramen [in Chinese], *Chin. J. Minim Invasive Neurosurg.* **24**(11), 522.

[10] Can H., Unal T.C., Dolas I., et al. (2020) Comprehensive anatomic and morphometric analyses of triangular working zone for transforaminal endoscopic approach in lumbar spine: A fresh cadaveric study, *World Neurosurg.* **138**, e486.

Chapter 4

V-Shape Bichannel Endoscopy Assisted Discectomy and Decompression

Section Editors:

Shisheng He, MD
Zhongliang Deng, MD
Haijian Ni, MD
Zhengjian Yan, MD
Jia Chen, MD

The third-generation spinal endoscopy system represented by YESS and TESSYS has greatly promoted the development of spinal minimally invasive surgery. Because of its merits including minimally invasive, effective, and simple, this uniportal and unichannel coaxial endoscopy technology shows great advantages in both discectomy and decompression in lateral spinal canal stenosis. The large spinal endoscopy system developed from these two techniques has increased the efficiency of procedures like decompression. In addition, the application of visual trephine has significantly upgraded techniques like foraminoplasty and decompression. The technique and instrument improvement has expanded the application of spinal endoscopic surgery. More and more spinal surgeries are expected to be completed *via* endoscopic surgery, rather than traditional open surgery. As a result, spinal endoscopic technique has to deal with some complicated situations. Currently, the conventional spinal endoscopy system shows insufficient flexibility and will still encounter difficulties in procedures like decompression of complicated cases. VBE system was invented under this background and showed unique advantages in decompression of complicated cases [1-5].

The cannula designed for decompression (with a diameter of 6.3 mm) is smaller than the cannula for fusion (with a diameter of 13.1 mm). The VBE decompression cannula is suitable for a complicated discectomy, decompression of spinal stenosis, removal of bone mass in the spinal canal, and other options. There are two types of VBE cannula for decompression. According to their design and function, we defined them as Type I and Type II. Details will be described in the following contents.

Like the conventional endoscopic lumbar surgery, adequate preoperative preparation should be made before the VBE assisted lumbar decompression surgery. Firstly, it is necessary to precisely diagnose and identify the responsible segment by analyzing the patient's history, physical examination, and imaging examination results including X-ray, computed tomography (CT), and magnetic resonance imaging (MRI). Secondly, anatomical variation of the lumbosacral nerve should be ruled out *via* magnetic resonance neurography (MRN). According to the literature, anatomical variation of lumbosacral nerve is not rare, and this nerve anatomical variation will increase the difficulty of operation, as well as the risk of nerve injury during endoscopic surgery. Meanwhile, the surgical path planning should be completed based on the imaging examination results before surgery. Also, the pain and psychological condition of the patients should be assessed to evaluate the patient's tolerance to pain and select a suitable anesthesia method. Local anesthesia is enough for most cases. However, epidural anesthesia or general anesthesia might be necessary for patients with severe pain, pain sensitization, low pain tolerance, obsessive–compulsive disorder, anxiety, and/or inability to maintain posture for a long time. In addition, communication and education are very important for the patient to understand the disease and treatment process. For example, patients should be informed of the possibility of recurrence of symptoms after discectomy or decompression, as well as postoperative treatment expectations [6–11].

4.1 Application of Type I V-Shape Bichannel Endoscopy Decompression Cannula in Lumbar Surgery

4.1.1 Structure of Type I VBE Decompression Cannula

Type I VBE decompression cannula (Figure 4.1) is designed for stable dorsal operation during the surgery, and is composed of a small channel (3.8 mm) on the dorsal side and a large channel (6.5 mm) on the ventral side. The dorsal side of lumbar foramen is the main operating area during foraminoplasty. We can remove the bone structures of the facet joint and ligamentum flavum for decompression spinal canal through this cannula. Even though we can visualize the dorsal structures *via* the conventional uniportal and unichannel coaxial endoscope, instruments have difficulty reaching the dorsal part without moving the endoscope and working cannula together. Due to the fact that the dorsal side of foramen is bone, and the ventral side is soft tissue, the endoscope and working cannula can easily slide during procedures like foraminoplasty. Therefore, the surgeon needs to frequently adjust the position of the working cannula very often, which is time-consuming and inefficient. When it comes to this situation, Type I decompression VBE cannula can be used for better foraminoplasty and decompression. The conventional endoscope (6.3 mm) can be introduced through the big channel (6.5 mm) at the ventral side to provide visualization, and instruments like trephine, high-speed bur, piezosurgery, forceps, and laminectomy punch can be introduced through the small channel (3.8 mm) to remove bone and ligament tissues. During the operation through the small channel, the front end of this cannula is directly against the posterior edge of the intervertebral disc. Thus, surgeons can finish the foraminoplasty and decompression without moving the endoscope and cannula frequently, which means the system is very stable while operating the dorsal part.

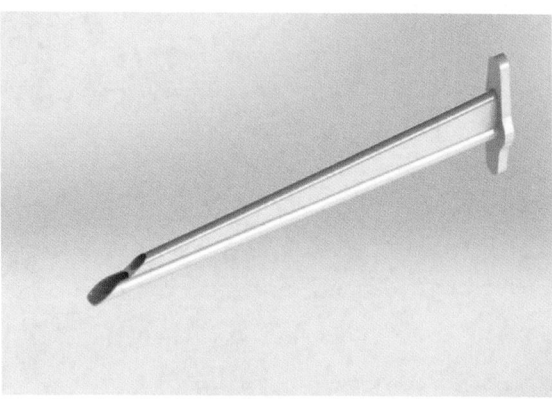

FIG. 4.1 Type I VBE working cannula for decompression.

4.1.2 Indications

Type I decompression VBE cannula is suitable for foraminoplasty and decompression for lateral spinal canal stenosis, which cannot reach satisfactory clinical outcomes with the conventional spinal endoscopic systems.

4.1.3 Instruments

Type I VBE decompression cannula, serial dilator, small visual trephine (or high-speed bur, piezosurgery), conventional spinal endoscopic system and associated instruments, light source, and imaging equipment.

4.1.4 Position

Both prone and lateral positions can be chosen based on the surgeon's habit.

4.1.5 Planning

The location, size, and migration of herniated disc tissue should be identified on imaging examination like MRI. The size of the intervertebral foramen and the height of the iliac crest should also be measured on X-ray image. Normally, the level of disc herniation is higher, the distance between puncture point and midline is smaller. For example, at L2/3 and L3/4, the distance from the puncture point to the midline is about 10 cm. This distance is longer at L4/5 and L5/S1, about 12–14 cm. Moreover, the distance from midline to the puncture point should be adjusted according to patient's body shape and obesity situation. For obese patients, this distance would be longer than normal. If the nucleus pulposus migrates downward, the entry point needs to be more cranial. The surface location of target segment, pedicle and foramen can be marked using a surface locator with X-ray. The outline of iliac crest can be drawn on the skin by palpation. Then, the puncture point and trajectory can be marked (Figure 4.2).

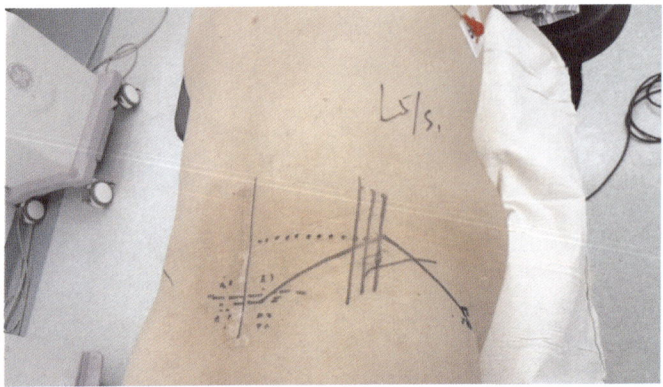

FIG. 4.2 The puncture point and trajectory.

4.1.6 Anesthesia

Local anesthesia is enough for most cases. However, epidural anesthesia or general anesthesia might be necessary for patients with severe pain, pain sensitization, low pain tolerance, obsessive–compulsive disorder, anxiety, and the inability to maintain posture for a long time. For local anesthesia, a sufficient block should be made under the skin, puncture path, and intervertebral foramen area. In addition, local anesthesia combined with intravenous sedation/analgesia is also a solution.

4.1.7 Establishment of Working Channel for Unichannel Endoscope System

After local anesthesia, an 18G hollow puncture needle is used to puncture through the intervertebral foramen. Then, the guidewire can be inserted, and serial dilation can be performed. The following procedure is foraminoplasty, which can be completed using a serial manual bone drill or trephine. X-ray is necessary to monitor the position of the bone drill or trephine. After the foraminoplasty is completed, conventional spinal endoscope can be introduced following the guidewire. The foraminoplasty effect can be evaluated under the endoscope view, and the Type I VBE decompression cannula can be used to further enlarge the foramen or decompress spinal canal if necessary.

4.1.8 Establishment of Working Channel for Type I VBE Decompression Cannula

A guidewire can be inserted through the conventional cannula to maintain the position. Then, after withdrawal of the conventional cannula, the Type I VBE decompression cannula can be introduced following the guidewire. Since the VBE cannula is larger than the conventional one, the skin incision should be extended for another 1–2 mm. After confirmation on X-ray, hammer the VBE cannula gently to anchor it into the ideal position (Figures 4.3 and 4.4). Normally, it will take about 30 seconds for this procedure.

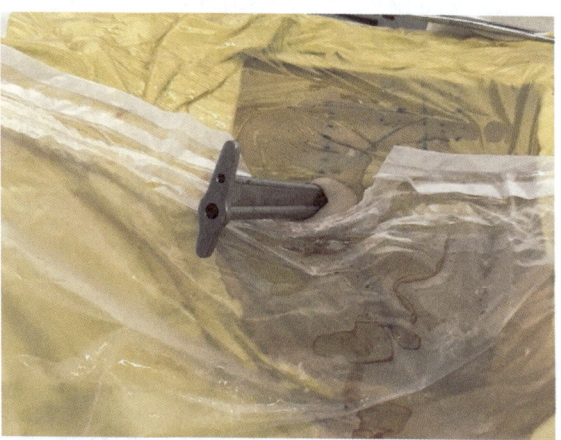

FIG. 4.3 Establishment of working channel for Type I VBE decompression cannula.

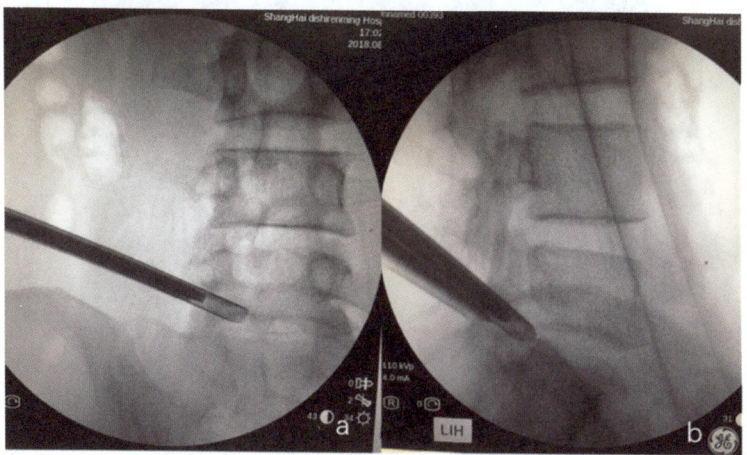

FIG. 4.4 Confirming the cannula's position on X-ray.
(a) Anteroposterior view; (b) lateral view.

4.1.9 *Foraminoplasty with Type I VBE Decompression Cannula*

A conventional spinal endoscope (6.3 mm) can be introduced through the large channel of the Type I VBE decompression cannula to visualize the facet joint and spinal canal. Trephine, high-speed bur, or piezosurgery can be used through the small channel (3.8 mm) to resect bone structures that block the path (Figure 4.5). Because surgeons can monitor the whole procedure under the endoscope, this operation is very safe (Figure 4.6). By rotating the cannula to the cranial or caudal side, surgeons can precisely and effectively remove the blockade.

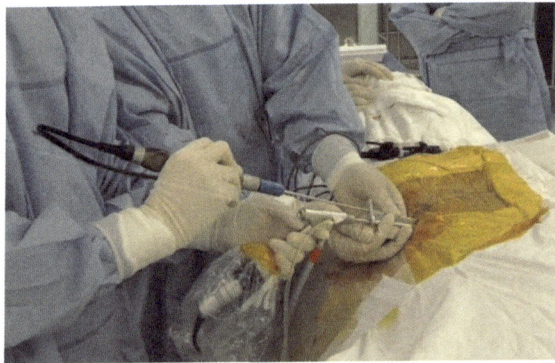

FIG. 4.5 Application of high-speed bur through the small channel of Type I VBE decompression cannula.

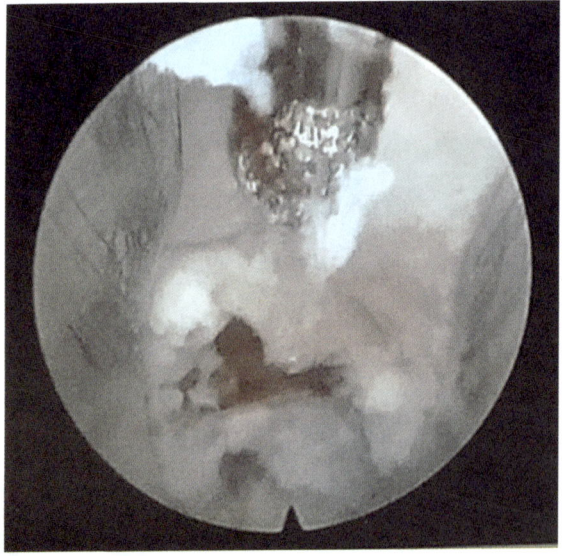

FIG. 4.6 Application of high-speed bur can be clearly monitored under the endoscope.

4.1.10 Discectomy and Decompression

The application of Type I VBE decompression cannula in discectomy and decompression is very flexible. The large channel of this cannula allows the application of the 6.3 mm conventional endoscope and associated instruments. Surgeons can also use instruments through the small channel to reach the dorsal part of the target field, which enlarges the operating range under the endoscopic view. What is more, instruments introduced through the two channels can cooperate with each other. For example, a nerve retractor can be introduced through one channel to protect the nerve root and dural sac, while discectomy and decompression can be performed through the other channel at the same time. Also, the switch between conventional cannula and VBE cannula is very convenient. In addition, the VBE cannula is very stable when dealing with dorsal tissue, which makes it suitable for removing ligamentum flavum and allowing for decompression in lateral spinal canal stenosis cases.

4.2 Application of Type II V-Shape Bichannel Endoscopy Decompression Cannula in Lumbar Surgery

4.2.1 Structure of Type II VBE Decompression Cannula

Type II VBE decompression cannula (Figure 4.7) is composed of a large channel (6.5 mm) on the dorsal side and a small channel (3.8 mm) on the ventral side. There is a specially designed endoscope with a diameter of 3.6 mm, which can be inserted through the small channel of Type II VBE decompression cannula to monitor the surgical field. The large channel is designed as the working channel, while the small channel is for visualization. Therefore, large size instruments can be used through the working channel to improve operation efficiency. The Type II VBE decompression cannula is designed for discectomy, foraminoplasty, and osteophyte excision. Because the whole procedure can be monitored under the endoscope, the surgery is safe and efficient. Since large instruments can be used through the working cannula, the resection of calcified disc tissue and bone structure is convenient. Compared with delicate endoscopic instruments, the large instruments used in the VBE technique are more solid and less likely to be damaged. As a result, the cost of instrument replacement is low. Unlike the Type I VBE decompression cannula, the Type II cannula has more working space for operation at the dorsal side. Even though the application of large instruments through the working cannula of Type II cannula can improve the operation efficiency, the special designed endoscope (3.6 mm) is necessary for visualization.

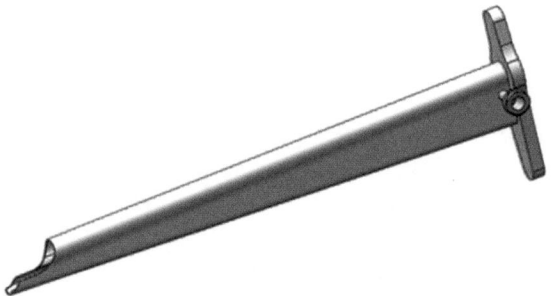

FIG. 4.7 Type II VBE decompression cannula.

4.2.2 Indications

Type II VBE decompression cannula can be used for discectomy, the resection of calcified disc tissue and osteophyte at the posterior edge of vertebral body. This cannula can also be used for difficult cases of foraminoplasty or decompression of lateral spinal canal stenosis.

4.2.3 *Instruments*

Type II VBE decompression cannula, inner core of the cannula, serial dilator, trephine and half-trephine, nerve retractor, water plugger, a specially designed endoscope with a diameter of 3.6 mm, large instruments designed for working channel, conventional spinal endoscopic system, and associated instruments, light source, and imaging equipment *et al*.

4.2.4 *Position*

Both prone and lateral positions can be chosen based on the surgeon's habits.

4.2.5 *Planning*

The surgical planning is similar to conventional endoscopic lumbar surgery. Imaging examinations like MRI, CT, and X-ray should be analyzed carefully to identify the location, calcification, size of the herniated disc tissue, and the site of spinal canal stenosis. The height of iliac crest, the variation of lumbosacral, the shape of foramen, and the hypertrophy of facet joint should also be analyzed during surgical planning. Normally, the level of disc herniation is higher, the distance between puncture point and midline is smaller. For example, at L2/3 and L3/4, the distance from puncture point to the midline is about 10 cm. This distance is longer at L4/5 and L5/S1, about 12–14 cm. At L5/S1 level, the puncture trajectory should tilt to the cranial side to avoid the iliac crest. Horizontal puncture trajectory would be suitable for higher level vertebrae. When the herniated mass migrates downward, the puncture trajectory should tilt to the caudal side.

4.2.6 *Anesthesia*

For patients without severe pain, low pain tolerance, or compulsivity, local anesthesia would be enough. Local anesthesia is very convenient and makes it possible for the surgeon to communicate with the patient during the surgery. Nerve irritation will cause the patient severe pain and alert the surgeon. Therefore, local anesthesia is a safe choice for endoscopic lumbar surgery. The main disadvantage of local anesthesia is that sometimes the analgesic effect can wear off. Once the patient cannot tolerate the pain, the surgery has to be terminated. What is more, severe pain might lead to elevated blood pressure and cardiovascular and cerebrovascular accidents. It is safer if anesthesiologists help in sedation and analgesia. The pain tolerance of patients can be evaluated before operation to judge whether local anesthesia is feasible. In addition, sedative and analgesic drugs can be used before the operation to improve the patient's tolerance of pain. For local anesthesia, a sufficient block should be made under the skin, puncture path, and intervertebral foramen area. Anesthesia in the intervertebral foramen area can be divided into two steps: local anesthesia around the facet joint and epidural anesthesia in the intervertebral foramen. Epidural anesthesia or general anesthesia might be necessary for patients with severe pain, pain sensitization, low pain tolerance, compulsive position, anxiety, and inability to maintain posture for the surgery.

4.2.7 The Establishment of the Working Cannula

After local anesthesia, a special puncture needle can be used to puncture through the intervertebral foramen. The ideal position of the needle tip is the ventral side of the facet joint bottom or the posterior superior edge of inferior vertebral body. Then, serial dilation can be performed. The Type II VBE decompression cannula can be introduced following the needle. After the confirmation of the position of the cannula on X-ray, the endoscope and monitor can be connected. After withdrawing the needle, the 3.6 mm endoscope can be introduced through the small channel of Type II VBE decompression cannula to visualize the surgical field. Radiofrequency electrode can be used to clean the soft tissue outside the intervertebral foramen and around the articular process to identify the anatomical structure around the foramen. Trephine or high-speed bur can be used to resect the facet joint to access the spinal canal. Then, structures like facet joints, ligamentum flavum, epidural space, herniated disc tissue, or other lesions can be clearly visualized *via* the endoscope. Gently tap the cannula until it reaches a satisfactory position.

4.2.8 Discectomy and Decompression

The length of traditional spinal surgery instruments like forceps and laminectomy punch can be increased and customized by the manufacturer. These instruments can be directly used through the large channel of Type II VBE decompression cannula to improve the operation efficiency, especially for calcified or sclerotic lesions. Also, the instrument is not easily damaged, and the operation is simpler and more flexible. If hemostasis is difficult, bone wax or gelatin sponge can be used when necessary. The nerve retractor and annular baffle can also be used through the large channel of the cannula to block nerves and other tissues, so as to avoid the damage of nerves and other important structures. In addition, the surgeon can also switch to conventional cannula and spinal endoscope (6.3 mm) for a follow-up procedure like decompression.

References

[1] Kanno H., Aizawa T., Hahimoto K., *et al.* (2019) Minimally invasive discectomy for lumbar disc herniation: Current concepts, surgical techniques, and outcomes, *Int. Orthop.* **43**(4), 917.
[2] Ahn Y. (2019) Endoscopic spine discectomy: Indications and outcomes, *Int. Orthop.* **43**(4), 909.
[3] Rasouli M.R., Rahimi-Movaghar V., Shokraneh F., *et al.* (2014) Minimally invasive discectomy versus microdiscectomy/open discectomy for symptomatic lumbar disc herniation, *Cochrane Database Syst. Rev.* (9), Cd010328.
[4] Akinduro O.O., Kerezoudis P., Alvi M.A., *et al.* (2017) Open versus minimally invasive surgery

for extraforaminal lumbar disk herniation: A systematic review and meta-analysis, *World Neurosurg.* **108**, 924.

[5] Xin G., Shi-Sheng H., Hai-Long Z. (2013) Morphometric analysis of the YESS and TESSYS techniques of percutaneous transforaminal endoscopic lumbar discectomy, *Clin. Anat.* **26**(6), 728.

[6] Burke S.M., Safain M.G., Kryzanski J., *et al.* (2013) Nerve root anomalies: Implications for transforaminal lumbar interbody fusion surgery and a review of the Neidre and Macnab classification system, *Neurosurg. Focus* **35**(2), E9.

[7] Song Q.P., Hai B., Zhao W.K., *et al.* (2021) Full-endoscopic foraminotomy with a novel large endoscopic trephine for severe degenerative lumbar foraminal stenosis at L(5) S(1) level: An advanced surgical technique, *Orthop. Surg.* **13**(2), 659.

[8] Chen C., Ma X., Zhao D., *et al.* (2021) Full endoscopic lumbar foraminoplasty with periendoscopic visualized trephine technique for lumbar disc herniation with migration and/or foraminal or lateral recess stenosis, *World Neurosurg.* **148**, e658.

[9] Jie L., WenboDiao, Yiming L., *et al.* (2019) Visual trephine for foraminoplasty in percutaneous endoscopic transforaminal discectomy, *Orthop. J. China* **27**(24), 2242.

[10] Simao S., Xiaom X., Dun W., *et al.* (2021) Effectiveness and safety of visualized trephine used in transforaminal endoscopy, *Orthop. J. China* **29**(1), 18.

[11] Zhu Y., Zhao Y., Fan G., *et al.* (2018) Comparison of 3 anesthetic methods for percutaneous transforaminal endoscopic discectomy: A prospective study, *Pain Physician* **21**(4), E347.

Chapter 5

V-Shape Bichannel Endoscopic Lumbar Fusion

Section Editors:

Shisheng He, MD
Jixian Qian, MD
Haijian Ni, MD
Chengpei Zhou, MD
Jia Chen, MD

Lumbar fusion has been proved to be a very effective method for the treatment of lumbar diseases through long-term clinical practice. Lumbar fusion technology is always developing. From interlaminar fusion, posterolateral fusion to interbody fusion, various technologies are becoming more and more mature, and the curative effect is more and more accurate. Minimally invasive lumbar fusion technology is welcomed by doctors and patients because of its small amount of trauma and rapid recovery. It is one of the hotspots in the development of spinal surgery in recent years [1, 2]. MIS-TLIF is a classic minimally invasive lumbar fusion technology, which has been widely used in clinics, and its curative effect has been proven effective in practice. Some new interbody fusion technologies such as ALIF/XLIF/OLIF have also been widely developed in clinics in recent years, and their effectiveness is also being tested. The total endoscopic lumbar interbody fusion technology is the least invasive and the most popular technology in the minimally invasive spinal fusion technology, and its surgical technology and related instruments are still gradually improving [3, 4].

At present, the clinical application of endoscopic lumbar interbody fusion technology can be divided into three categories: uniportal and unichannel coaxial endoscopy (including wide channel endoscopy) assisted lumbar interbody fusion, unilateral bichannel endoscopy (UBE) assisted lumbar interbody fusion, and MED assisted lumbar interbody fusion.

Uniportal and unichannel coaxial endoscope such as the conventional "intervertebral foraminal endoscope", includes the wide channel endoscope. It can remove the articular process or part of the vertebral lamina and articular process through the endoscopic tool or external visual trephine. Therefore, it can reach the spinal canal through the intervertebral foramen approach or the posterior approach to complete the interbody fusion operation similar to TLIF or PLIF. However, due to the current working channel diameter of coaxial endoscope, these instruments for conventional open surgery and interbody fusion cage cannot be placed through the tail end of the channel. Therefore, after the treatment of the intervertebral space, it is necessary to exit the endoscope and replace it with a channel with a larger diameter, and complete interbody model testing, fusion cage placement and other steps under repeated fluoroscopy confirmation. These steps do not have the whole process of monitoring using the endoscope. The possibility of nerve injury cannot be avoided, so it can only be called "endoscopic assisted" interbody fusion [5].

The characteristic of UBE technology is that the endoscope and working channel are completely independent, forming an operation mode similar to arthroscopy, so as to expand the field of vision. At the same time, conventional open surgical instruments can be used in the working channel. However, this technology mainly passes through the posterior approach, which needs to remove a part of the vertebral lamina and a part of the articular process like open surgery, and properly pull the dural sac inward, Therefore, epidural hematocele and long-term dural adhesion cannot be avoided, and the injury to lumbar muscles caused by the repeated entry and exit of surgical instruments during the operation cannot be ignored. That being said, it is worth discussing whether the UBE technology is the real "most minimally invasive" [6-10].

MED was applied in clinics in the 1990s, but due to the lack of understanding by clinicians, poor imaging effect at that time, and frequent wiping due to surgical smoke and blood accumulation on the lens, this technology remained silent for nearly ten years. With the development of spinal minimally invasive technology, MED has been applied again by some spinal minimally invasive surgeons. In the future, with the continuous improvement of imaging system and the advent of some improved products (such as MED in aqueous medium), MED technology will have better application prospects.

VBE lumbar fusion technology is a new endoscopic lumbar interbody fusion technology based on VBE endoscopic system. Its surgical approach is similar to MIS-TLIF surgery. It can also be understood as a VBE endoscopic system to complete interbody fusion through intervertebral foramen, namely "VBE-TLIF". Therefore, this technology directly enters the intervertebral disc through Kambin's triangle by cutting off a part of the articular process. The operation path is direct and fast, with little disturbance to the dural sac and nerve root. The whole operation is carried out under the monitoring of VBE endoscope, without repeated fluoroscopy. The operation is safe, reliable, simple, and easy.

5.1 Anatomy

VBE lumbar fusion technology directly enters the intervertebral disc by removing part of the facet joints in the Kambin triangle. The lower facet of the lumbar facet joint is on the inside, and the upper facet is on the outside. The upper facet is mainly removed when the facet joint is removed. Sometimes part of the lower facet needs to be removed. If there is lateral stenosis, more joints, ligamentum flavum and lamina can be removed on the inside as needed. The medial boundary of the Kambin triangle is the dural sac and the lateral edge of the inferior is the traversing root. The bottom edge is the upper endplate of the inferior vertebral body, and the oblique edge is the exiting nerve root. There are no nerves in this area, and there are few arteriovenous vessels, so it is relatively safe to enter the intervertebral space. The top of the intervertebral foramen is the subarachnoid notch of the upper vertebral body. The bottom is the subarachnoid notch of the lower vertebral body. The front boundary is the posterior edge of the adjacent vertebral body and the intervertebral disc, and the rear boundary is the upper and lower articular processes. The inner side is the dural sac and the lower traversing root, and the outer side is the iliopsoas muscle. The upper and lower diameter of lumbar intervertebral foramen generally decreases from top to bottom, and L5/S1 is the smallest. The anterior posterior diameter is relatively constant, generally less than the upper and lower diameter, but the anterior posterior diameter of L5/S1 intervertebral foramen can be greater than the upper and lower diameter. The intervertebral foramen of L1–4 is keyhole shaped, and the intervertebral foramen of L5/S1 is oval. There are spinal branches of spinal nerve, lymphatic vessel and segmental artery in the intervertebral foramen (divided into 3 branches after entering the intervertebral foramen, which supply nerve, intraspinal tissue and posterior vertebral body respectively), communicating vein between intraspinal and extravertebral venous plexus, 2–4 sinus vertebral nerves and adipose tissue. From the midline to the outside of the lumbar intervertebral foramen, the superior nerve root gradually moves downward, and the more to the outside, and moves closer and closer to the intervertebral disc [11, 12].

The incidence of nerve root variation is 1.3%–14%. If there is nerve root variation during lumbar surgery, it will significantly increase the risk of nerve injury, especially in minimally invasive lumbar fusion surgery. The most common nerve root variation occurs in L5/S1. The intraoperative discovery rate of surgeons was about 1.3%, the discovery rate of MRI and myelography CT scanning was about 2.2%–4%, and the discovery rate reported by autopsy was 8.5%–14%. Neidre Classification of nerve root variation is commonly used. Type I: the most common. The nerve roots go out from their intervertebral foramen, but the position is abnormal. Type IA: one nerve root is sent from the dura mater, and then divided into two. Type IB: two nerve roots are sent out from the dura mater, but the two nerve roots are too close to each other. Type II: two nerve roots go out from one intervertebral foramen. Type IIA: two nerve roots in one intervertebral foramen and zero nerve roots in the other intervertebral foramen. Type IIB: two nerve roots in one intervertebral foramen and one nerve root in the other intervertebral foramen. Type III: anastomotic branches exist between adjacent nerve roots. Therefore, careful analysis should be carried out before minimally invasive lumbar fusion to understand nerve root deformity [13, 14].

From the analysis of X-ray, CT, MRI and MRN, the abduction angle of VBE is mostly between 30° and 45°. Generally, the best side opening distance is 6–9 cm. L5/S1 is affected by the iliac crest, so the lateral opening distance is smaller, and the lateral opening distance of L4/5 is relatively large. At more cranial levels, the ideal entry point is less distant from the midline.

5.2 Surgical Instruments and Equipment

Surgical instruments include 14 mm VBE bichannel working cannula, puncture guide needle, step-by-step expansion tool, various trephine (ordinary trephine, trephine with internal threads, trephine with internal threads that can be tightened, semi trephine), water blocking, nerve retractor used under endoscopy, suction tube used under endoscopy, lengthened front and back mouth gun forceps that can be used in routine surgery, nucleus pulposus forceps, intervertebral distractor, intervertebral space treatment reamer, curettage spoon, bone graft funnel, fusion cage implantation tools, and working cannula, nucleus pulposus forceps, gun forceps, RF electrode used under conventional unichannel intervertebral foraminal endoscope, etc. Two endoscopes are prepared for surgery, one is a 3.6 mm VBE endoscope, and the other is a 6.3 mm conventional intervertebral foraminal endoscope. There is also imaging equipment, power equipment, RF equipment and a percutaneous pedicle screw system. If possible, neurophysiological monitoring equipment can also be used.

5.3 Layout of Operating Room

The patient is placed on the fluoroscopic operating table. There is no barrier between the lower part of the operating table from the waist to the head and the ground, which does not affect the fluoroscopy of the lumbar surgical site. The C-arm X-ray machine can move freely from the waist to the head, which is convenient for intraoperative fluoroscopy. When the C-arm X-ray machine is adjusted to the appropriate position, it can obtain a satisfactory positive and lateral position. After that, the C-arm can be moved to the head side without fluoroscopy, and then to the operation site when fluoroscopy is needed, so as to save the operation time. The C-arm X-ray machine can be placed on the opposite side of the operation side or on the same side, and the display device and RF machine can be placed on the opposite side of the operation. In order to facilitate the collection of a large amount of flushing fluid during the operation, the exclusive collection water bag of arthroscopy can be used (Figure 5.1).

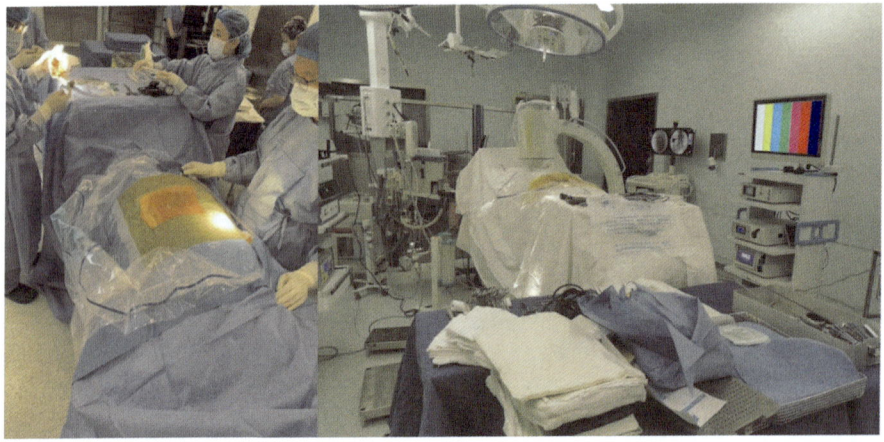

FIG. 5.1 VBE operating room layout arrangement.

5.4 Surgical Indications

VBE lumbar fusion is applicable to all patients who need fusion except for severe lumbar central spinal canal stenosis. For patients who need only one side decompression and fusion, VBE decompression and fusion through one side approach can be adopted. For patients who need bilateral decompression, VBE decompression and fusion through one side approach and endoscopic decompression on the other side can be adopted.

The main indications include:

(1) Lumbar spinal stenosis dominated by lateral stenosis
(2) Lumbar spondylolisthesis
(3) Lumbar instability
(4) Recurrent lumbar disc herniation requires interbody fusion
(5) Discogenic low back pain
(6) Giant lumbar disc herniation

For patients with recurrent and giant disc herniation, whether the lumbar fusion is required needs careful consideration. Generally, only minimally invasive removal of the protruding nucleus pulposus is required, but these patients may eventually have to undergo lumbar fusion surgery. Minimally invasive surgery can delay the time of fusion and even avoid fusion.

5.5 Surgical Contraindications

(1) Patients with severe osteoporosis
(2) Nerve root variation in the fusion segment, which is not suitable for patients with interbody fusion
(3) Severe central spinal stenosis
(4) Severe lumbar spondylolisthesis above grade III
(5) Infection in intervertebral space and adjacent parts
(6) Patients with other diseases affecting fusion or unable to tolerate surgery

5.6 Surgical Methods

5.6.1 Preoperative Preparation and Planning

It is necessary to carefully ask the patient's medical history, do physical examination and auxiliary examination before operation, clarify the patient's diagnosis, and consider whether to choose VBE operation after eliminating relevant contraindications. Before operation, read the X-ray film carefully to analyze for rotation of the vertebral body, scoliosis, joint hyperplasia, presence or absence of transitional vertebra and other spinal variations. The height of intervertebral space, the size and height of the intervertebral foramen and the condition of diseased intervertebral facets can be observed through the lateral film (Figure 5.2). The three-dimensional morphology of the intervertebral foramen and lumbar spine can be observed through the three-dimensional reconstruction CT. Carefully analyze the sagittal and transverse scanning of lumbar MRI, observe whether there is variation in the nerve root of the surgical segment, master the course of the nerve root, plan the surgical path and precautions, and avoid damaging the nerve (Figures 5.3 and 5.4). According to the planned surgical path, measure the lateral opening distance and angle of puncture on lumbar MRI. Generally, the lateral opening distance of lumbar VBE is between 6 and 9 cm. The closer to the head, the smaller the lateral opening distance, and the camber angle is generally between 30° and 45°.

5.6.2 Body Position and Surface Location

The patient is in the prone position with the abdomen suspended. If possible, neuroelectrophysiological monitoring can be used. Mark the position of the pedicle screw and the position of the double channel endoscopic incision with the body surface locator on the body surface (Figure 5.5). Routinely disinfect and lay operation sheet. Because the dual channel endoscope needs two channels of flushing water, it is necessary to prepare an extra 3000 ml flushing water and heat the flushing water at the same time to avoid too much flushing water affecting the patient's body temperature. Use the water bag of arthroscopy to collect the irrigation liquid, and plan the position of C-arm machine and imaging equipment in advance to facilitate surgical operation and fluoroscopy and avoid repeated adjustment and delay of the operation time.

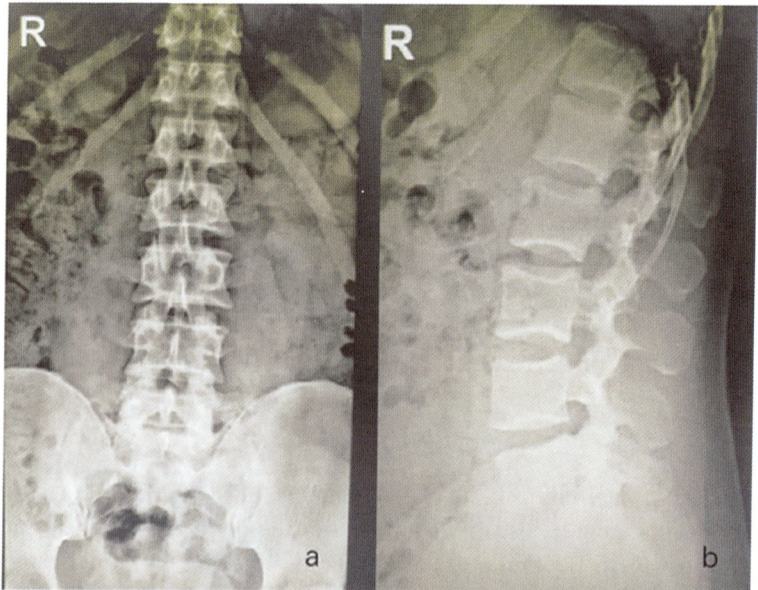

FIG. 5.2 X-ray image of lumbar spine.
(a) Anteroposterior view; (b) lateral view.

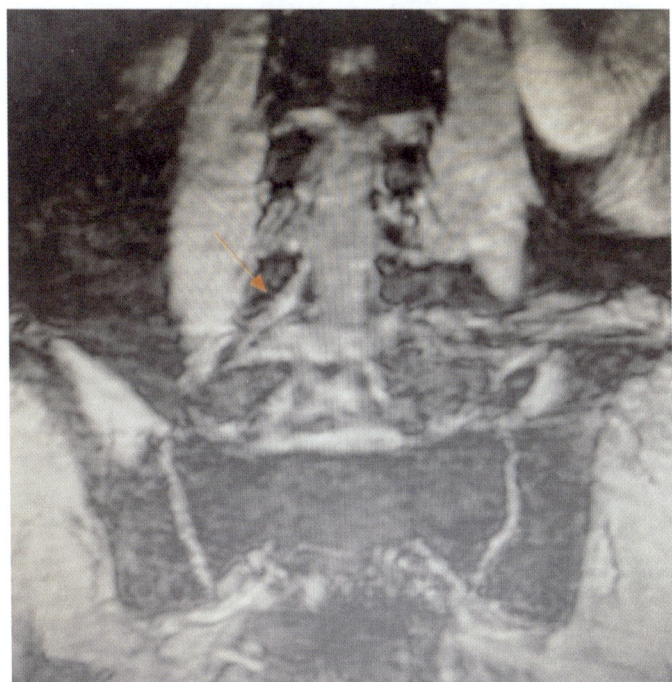

FIG. 5.3　Lumbar magnetic resonance neuroimaging.

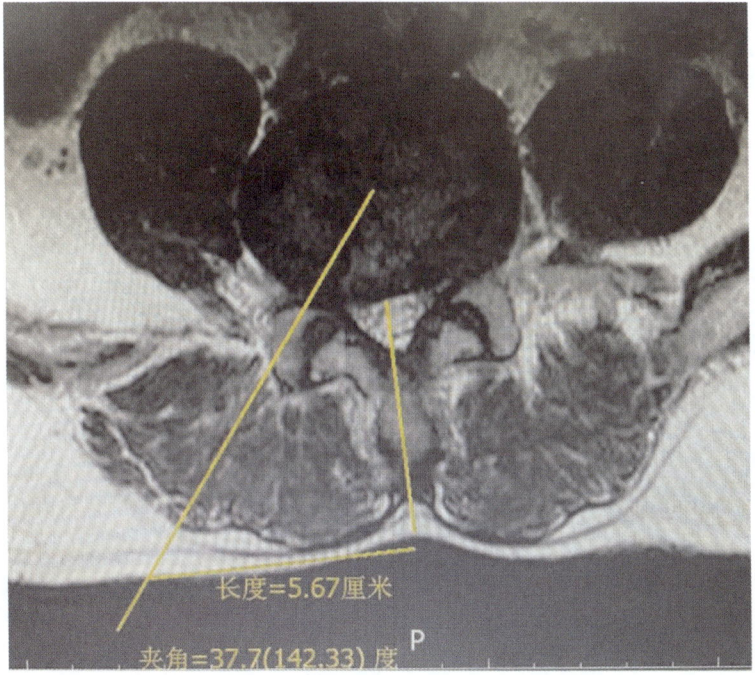

FIG. 5.4　Lumbar MRI axial scan.

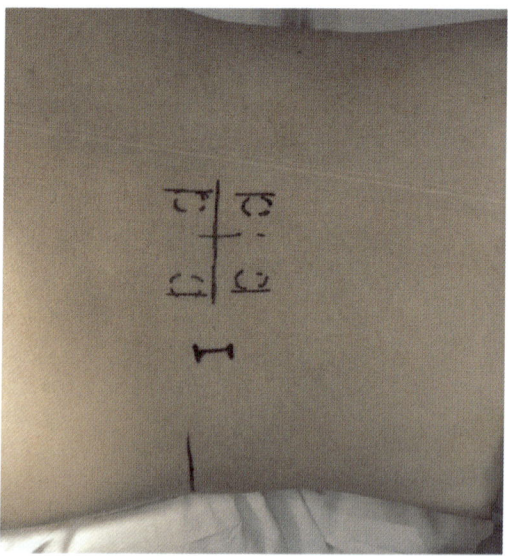

FIG. 5.5 Body surface positioning of pedicle screws and location of bichannel endoscopic incision.

5.6.3 *Operation Process*

(1) Placement of guide wire for percutaneous pedicle screw

Generally, the guide wire of the segment requiring percutaneous pedicle screw fixation is placed under fluoroscopy. The endoscopic fusion can also be carried out first, and then the percutaneous pedicle screw guide wire can be placed and fixed.

(2) Placement of puncture needle

There are special blunt and pointed puncture needles in the supporting instruments, which can be selected according to the preferences of surgeons. The best puncture path is along the superior endplate of the lower vertebral body, close to the lateral edge of the facet joint, and penetrated at an angle of about 45°. It is easy to hurt the exiting root on the upper and outer side, while it is easy to hurt the dural sac and traversing root on the inner side. Therefore, we should carefully read the imaging data before operation, plan the preoperative path, and determine the best puncture path (Figures 5.6 and 5.7).

(3) Establishment of working cannula

When the position of the puncture needle is appropriate, use the corresponding expansion tube to expand step by step. During expansion, pay attention to whether the puncture needle is displaced. In particular, be careful that the puncture needle cannot be brought to the front and damage the blood vessels in the front and organs in the abdominal cavity. After the expansion, insert the working cannula with the inner core along the puncture needle. The cannula should be close to the facet joint. Often, the tip of

Chapter 5 V-Shape Bichannel Endoscopic Lumbar Fusion 63

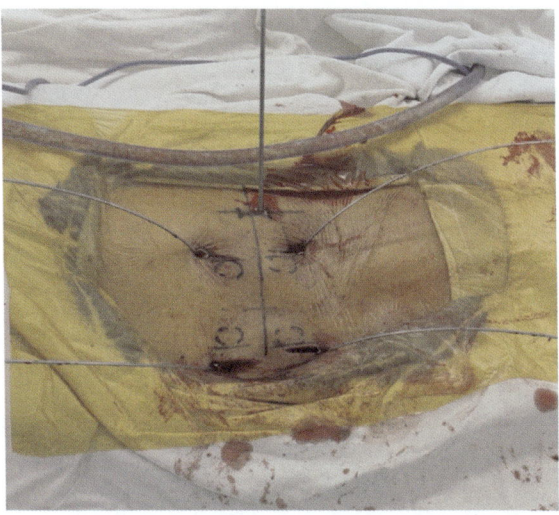

FIG. 5.6 Placement of guide wire and puncture needle.

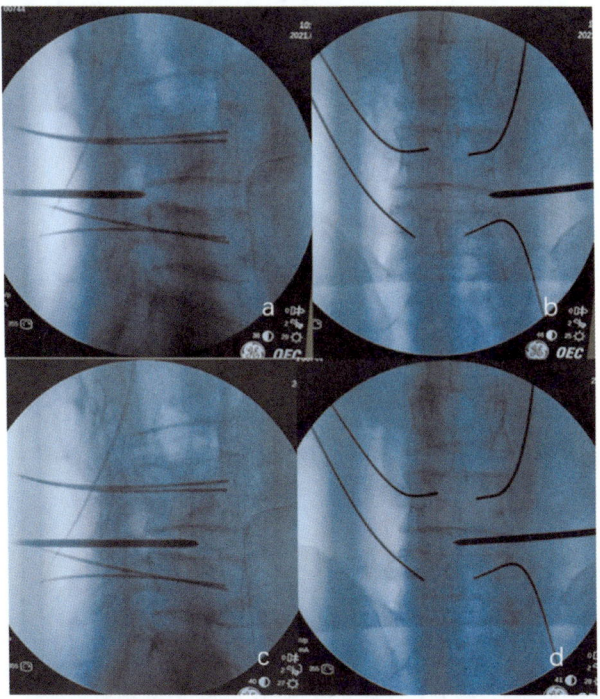

FIG. 5.7 C-arm fluoroscopy of guide wire and puncture needle placement.
(a), (b) Lateral view and anteroposterior view confirmed the puncture direction was good; (c), (d) the needle was punctured into the disc following that direction.

the cannula has reached the trailing edge of the intervertebral disc and is facing the intervertebral disc. It can be used as a positioning reference mark of the intervertebral disc under endoscopy (Figures 5.8 and 5.9). At this time, use the common trephine into the facet joint from the channel under direct vision or perspective (Figure 5.10). The lateral position of the trephine under perspective shall not exceed the ventral side of the small joint. If it exceeds the ventral side, be careful not to damage the exiting nerve root. The positive perspective trephine shall not exceed the inner edge of the pedicle, and if it exceeds the medial edge, be careful to not damage the traversing root and dural sac (Figure 5.11). After the trephine reaches the deepest safe position, if the bone block is not completely sawed off, you can shake the trephine and cannula up and down, left and right to split and break the bone block. After taking out the ordinary trephine, use the trephine with internal thread, hold the bone block, and then take it out (Figure 5.12). If the removal of the bone block is not smooth enough, it can be sawed in with a tightening ring saw, and then you can tighten the ring saw to take out the bone block. For some patients, it is difficult to take out the bone block. The main reason is that the root and inner side of the upper articular process of the lower vertebral body are not sawn off. At this time, the root of the upper articular process can be sawn off with a semi trephine under fluoroscopy or direct vision, and then the sawn bone block can be pried off. In the process of sawing, fluoroscopy is still needed to avoid the injury of the traversing root and dural sac. The bone blocks that are difficult to be removed with the ring saw can be taken out directly under the endoscope with the nucleus pulposus forceps, or taken out directly with the nucleus pulposus forceps, like MED after the water in the channel is sucked clean. The removed bone block needs to be preserved for bone grafting. If you are worried that the trephine will damage the nerve, you do not have to completely cut off the facet joints. The remaining facet joints can be directly taken off with laminectomy punch under endoscopic monitoring.

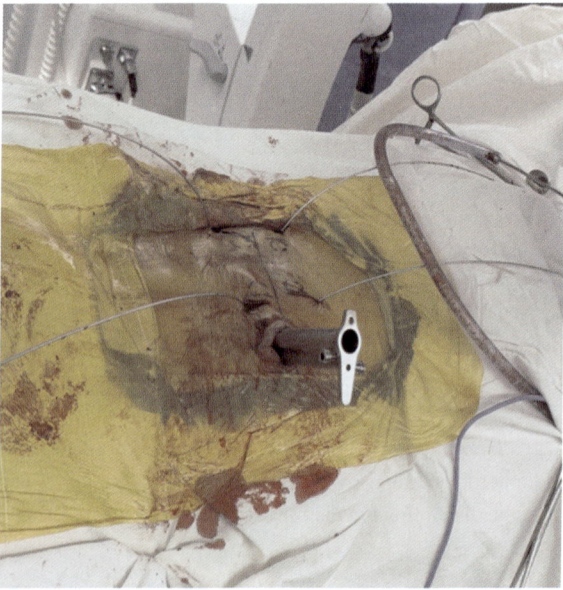

FIG. 5.8 The placement of VBE working cannula.

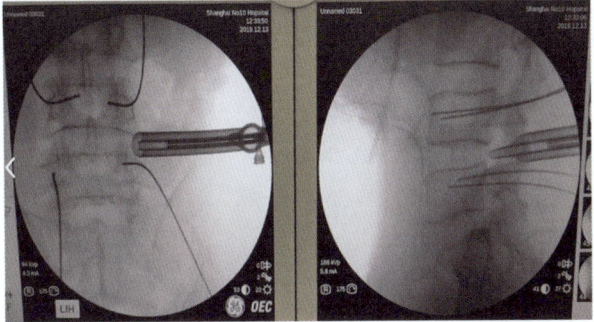

FIG. 5.9 Confirmation of VBE cannula by C-arm fluoroscopy.

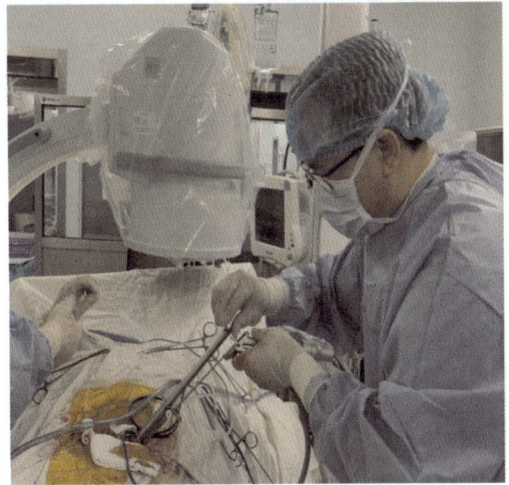

FIG. 5.10 Intraoperative image of saw in facet joint.

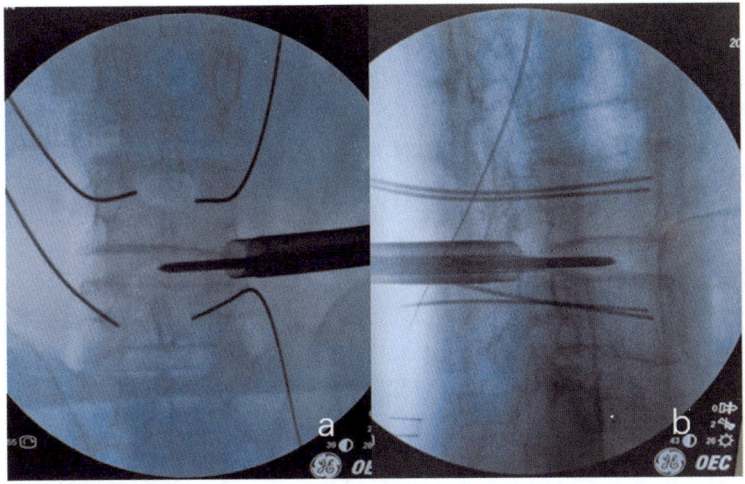

FIG. 5.11 Deepest safety position of trephine on X-ray.
(a) Anteroposterior view; (b) lateral view.

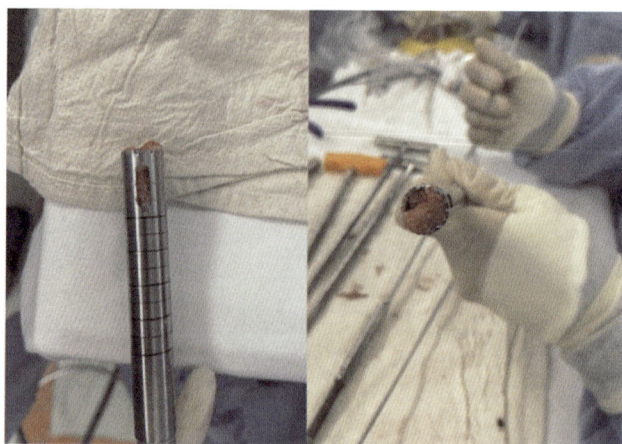

FIG. 5.12 The resected bone tissue.

(4) Intervertebral space treatment

After the bone block is removed by trephine and laminectomy punch, it can reach the intervertebral space directly. If the position of the intervertebral space cannot be well defined, the intervertebral space can be pricked with a Kirschner Pin under endoscopic monitoring, or the position of the intervertebral space can be confirmed through fluoroscopy. The subsequent intervertebral space treatment and operation are the same as the operation steps of conventional surgery. After lengthening, various conventional surgical instruments can be used under VBE endoscopy. Various conventional surgical instruments such as nucleus pulposus forceps are used to remove nucleus pulposus. Intervertebral space distractor is used, and intervertebral space reamer and scraper are used to deal with the endplate until blood seepage. The endplate should be protected (Figures 5.13 and 5.14). When dealing with the intervertebral space, pay attention to the depth and scale of the intervertebral space treatment instrument to prevent the instrument from being too deep and damaging the important blood vessels and organs on the ventral side. At present, the VBE microscopic tools were designed with depth limit, and the deepest entry into the intervertebral space will not exceed 40 mm, so as to ensure that the blood vessels and organs in front of the vertebral body will not be injured. At the same time, pay attention to the upper exiting nerve root and the medial dural sac and traversing root under endoscopy. If the above structures are found nearby, readjust the channel position or pull it away with a retractor to avoid nerve and dural sac injury.

(5) Bone grafting

After the treatment of the intervertebral space, insert the bone graft funnel into the intervertebral space for bone grafting. Pay attention to confirming the depth of the bone graft funnel to avoid injury to the front blood vessels and abdominal organs, and prevent the bone graft funnel from not inserted into the intervertebral space, as this would result in the implantation of bone blocks outside the intervertebral space. Interbody bone grafting needs to ensure sufficient bone grafting. Often the excised articular process autologous bone cannot meet the amount required for fusion. At this time, it is necessary to implant enough substitute materials, such as allogeneic bone or artificial bone, or add materials to promote bone formation such as BMP, so as to ensure the fusion of bone grafting.

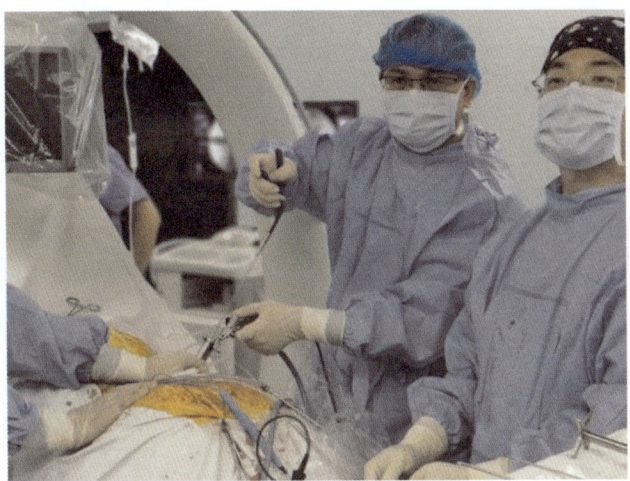

FIG. 5.13   ntraoperative image of intervertebral space treatment.

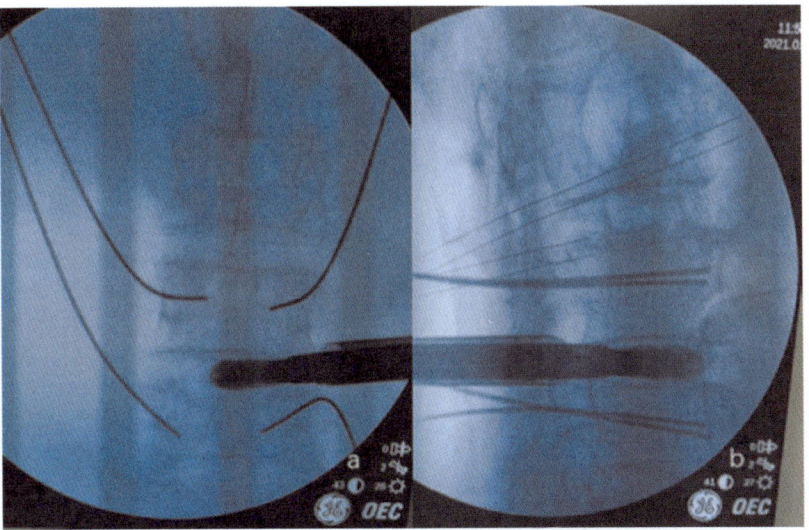

FIG. 5.14   C-arm fluoroscopy of intervertebral space treatment.

(6) Implantation of fusion cage

After bone grafting, the fusion cage was implanted. Under the VBE dual channel, the whole implantation process of the fusion cage can be carried out under endoscopic monitoring (Figure 5.15). According to the author's experience, because the bottom edge of the Kambin Triangle has a certain width (there is a certain distance between the exiting root and the traversing root in the intervertebral disc plane), in most cases, the fusion cage can be implanted simply through the Kambin Triangle by removing the articular process without disturbing the medial dural sac and nerve root.

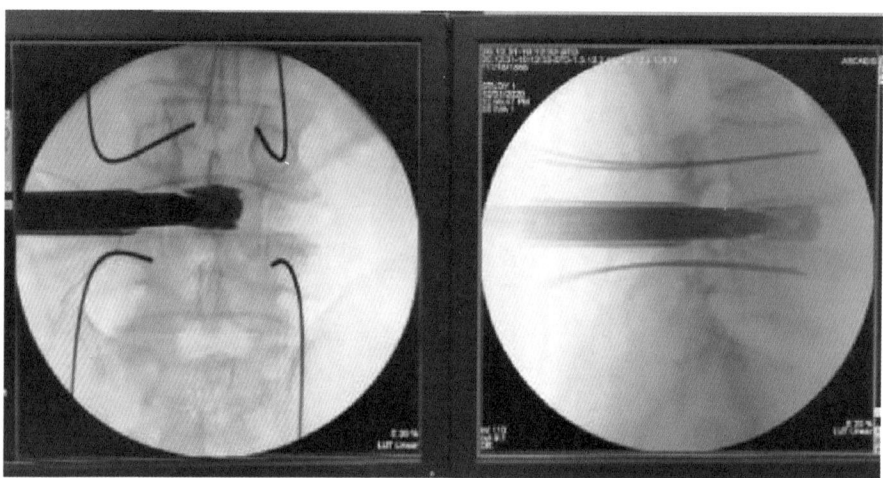

FIG. 5.15 C-arm fluoroscopy of fusion cage implantation.

(7) Ipsilateral and contralateral decompression

It is generally recommended to do decompression after the implantation of the fusion cage. Instead of replacing the working cannula, the dual channel instrument used for fusion can be directly used for decompression. If the field of vision is not very clear due to bleeding, the conventional intervertebral foraminal endoscope can be used for decompression and intervertebral discectomy. If there is intervertebral disc protrusion or stenosis on the opposite side, conventional intervertebral foraminal endoscopy can be used to decompress and remove the nucleus pulposus on the opposite side. The operations on both sides can be operated by two operators at the same time, which will not increase the operation time (Figures 5.16–5.21).

(8) Percutaneous pedicle screw fixation

After fusion and decompression, fix the percutaneous pedicle screw. After fluoroscopy and confirmation, insert the percutaneous screw along the placed guide wire, and then close the incision (Figures 5.22 and 5.23).

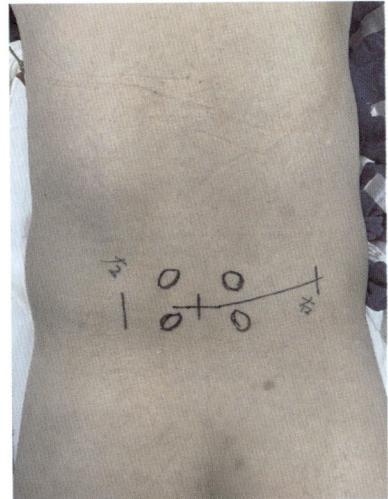

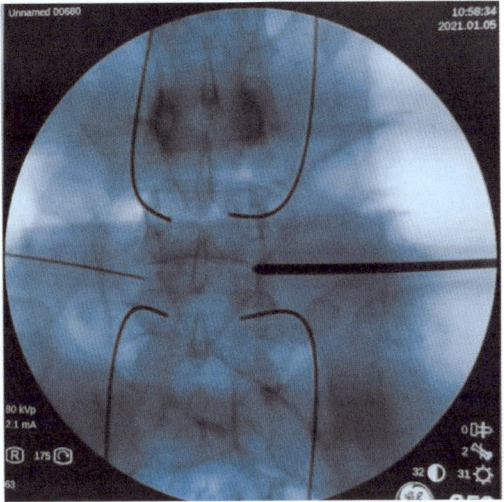

FIG. 5.16 Preoperative body surface positioning.

FIG. 5.17 Right VBE surgical path puncture, left conventional foraminal endoscopic path puncture.

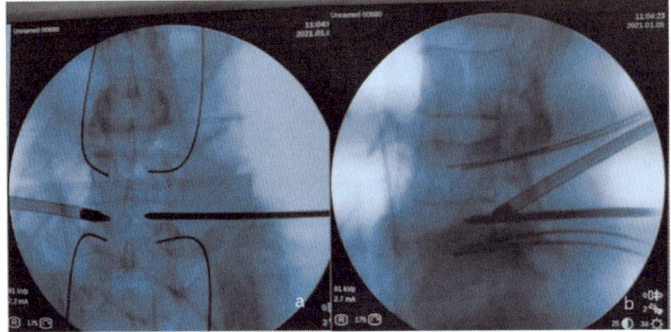

FIG. 5.18 Step by step expansion after fluoroscopy confirmed the puncture position on both sides.

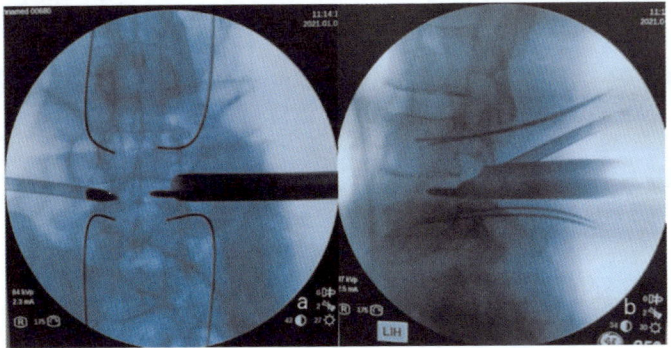

FIG. 5.19 Working cannula placed on both sides for bilateral decompression and unilateral fusion.

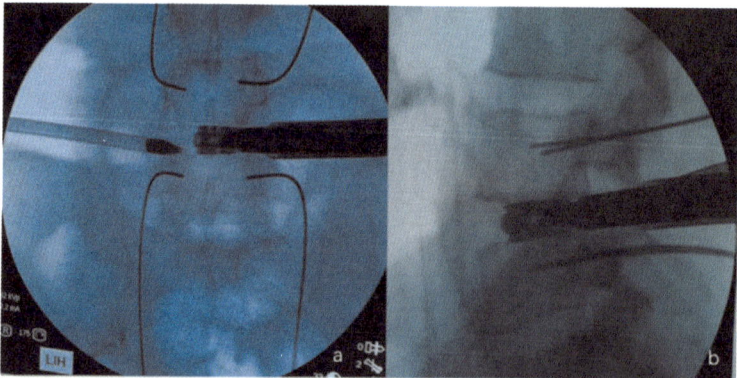

FIG. 5.20 Interbody bone grafting on VBE decompression and fusion side.

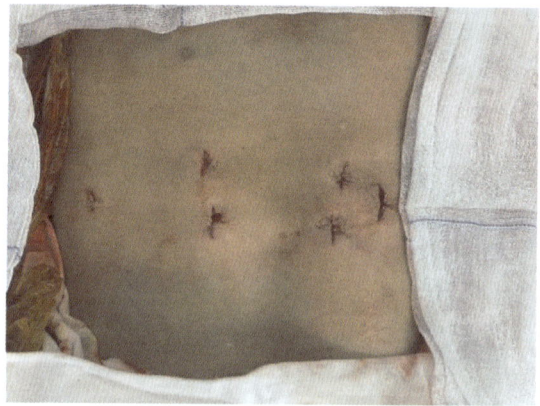

FIG. 5.21 Surgical incision.

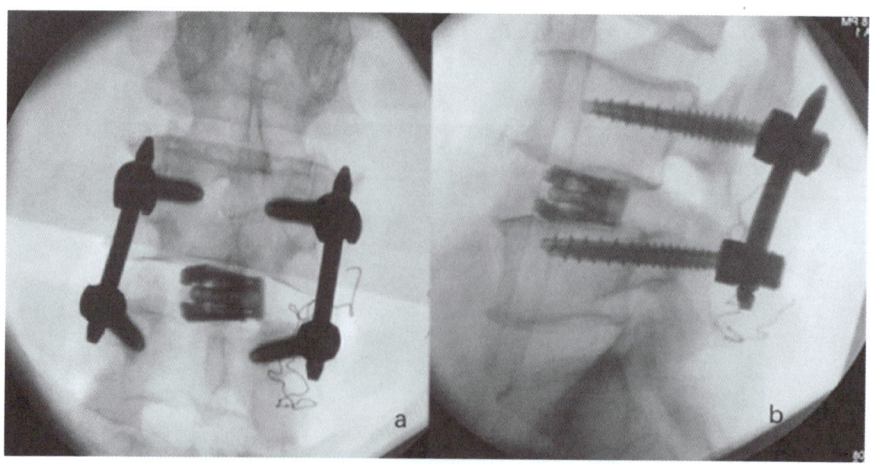

FIG. 5.22 C-arm fluoroscopy of percutaneous screw fixation.
(a) Anteroposterior view; (b) lateral view.

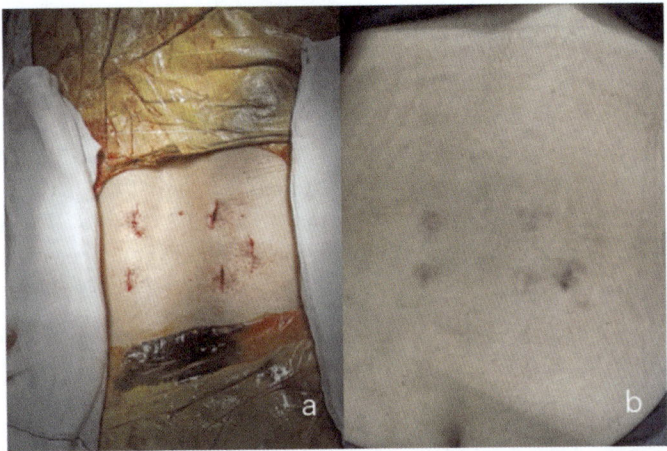

FIG. 5.23 Post percutaneous screw surgery.
(a) Surgical incision during the surgery; (b) 3 months after the surgery.

5.7 Precautions for Operation

5.7.1 Preoperative Imaging Data Analysis and Surgical Planning

Preoperative imaging data analysis is very important. We should carefully analyze X-ray film, CT, MRI, MRN and other data, eliminate bone and nerve root malformations, understand nerve direction, and avoid nerve injury. If there is nerve root deformity, it is often difficult to complete the interbody fusion on the deformity side. If there is pedicle deformity, percutaneous pedicle screw fixation cannot be completed. Before operation, the surgical path and incision location need to be planned according to the analysis of imaging data.

5.7.2 Direction of Puncture

The guide wire needs to be parallel to the intervertebral space and close to the upper end plate of the lower vertebral body. The position of the guide wire is very important. It is easy to damage the exiting root if it is too lateral (outside) and superior (upper), and it is easy to damage the dural sac and traversing root if it is too medial (inner). The guide wire needs to be parallel to the intervertebral space to facilitate the implantation of the fusion cage.

5.7.3 Location of Working Cannula

The working channel should be close to the facet joint, and the tip should be aligned with the posterior edge of the intervertebral disc, so as to facilitate the treatment of the intervertebral space and the implantation of the fusion cage. If it deviates, it will be difficult to operate. The tip of the working channel is a mark of the intervertebral space under the endoscope. The intervertebral disc is at the tip. It is very easy to identify under the endoscope. If it is difficult to find the intervertebral space under the endoscope, the working cannula may be displaced. Under the working channel, if the nerve root is not blocked, you need to readjust the working channel to block the nerve root, so as to ensure that there is no nerve in the operation area and the operation is safe. It is very important to maintain the correct position of the working channel, so that the path of removing the bone block is also suitable for the implantation of the fusion cage. If it deviates, there will be bone block on the path of the implantation of the fusion cage, which needs to be resected.

5.7.4 How to Use a Trephine to Remove Bones?

The depth of bone removal by trephine shall not exceed the ventral side of the small joint, otherwise it is easy cause injury to the exiting root of the intervertebral foramen. The inner side shall not exceed the inner edge of the pedicle, otherwise it is easy to cause injury the dural sac and traversing root. In order to avoid nerve injury, the trephine may not be able to completely cut the bone block. At this time, the trephine can be shaken up, down, left and right to split and break the bone block. When the root of the superior articular process cannot be sawn off, it can be sawn off with a semi trephine under direct vision, which can better avoid the injury of the exiting nerve root. You can try to take out the bone block with a threaded trephine and a tightening trephine with internal thread. If you still cannot take it out, you can take out the bone block directly with nucleus pulposus forceps or take it with gun forceps.

5.7.5 Hemostasis

Hemostasis under large channel endoscopy is sometimes difficult. At this time, it can be compressed with gelatin sponge to stop bleeding. One advantage of the VBE design is that it is compatible with MED. Turning off and flushing the water in the channel is the same as with MED. It can stop bleeding directly with bipolar electrocoagulation or long handle electric knife under endoscopic monitoring.

5.7.6 To Ensure the Fusion of Bone Graft

The endplate should be well protected. At the same time, it should be cleaned from blood on the bone surface. Try to take more autologous bone for bone grafting. When the bone volume is not enough, allogeneic bone or autologous bone should be implanted. BMP and other factors that promote bone formation can also be used.

5.7.7 Use of Water Plug

VBE has designed different shapes of water plug. The main function of water plug is to narrow the working channel and change the water flow, so that the flushing water can rush to the bottom of the channel to make the field of vision clearer. The function of the working channel can also adjust the position of instruments and work.

5.7.8 Precautions of Decompression

Use the VBE channel to accomplish the implantation of lumbar fusion cage. Operation under the VBE channel has the advantages of fast, efficient, whole-process visualization and safety. After bone graft fusion, if nucleus pulposus extraction and lateral spinal canal decompression are required, the large channel can be used. If the visual field is not very clear, the conventional intervertebral foraminal endoscope can be replaced for decompression.

5.7.9 Management of Working Cannula Shift

If the working cannula shifts during operation and the accurate position cannot be determined, the position can be reconfirmed through fluoroscopy.

5.7.10 Avoidance of Vascular Injury

When dealing with the intervertebral space, pay extra attention to the depth of the tool entering the intervertebral space to avoid vascular damage in front of the vertebral body. The current intervertebral space treatment tools are limited in depth. When the end handle of the instrument touches the end of the endoscope, the instrument enters the intervertebral space about 40 mm, and there are depth marks on the head and tail sides of the working channel. When operating under endoscope, pay attention to the depth of entry to prevent damage to the blood vessels and organs in front.

5.8 Postoperative Treatment

VBE lumbar interbody fusion has less bleeding. Generally, drainage should not be placed after the operation. Patients can decrease waist circumference 2–3 days after the operation. Patients should carry out low back muscle exercise and straight leg lifting exercise in bed. Patients can gradually recover daily activities in about three weeks.

5.9 Prevention of Complications

5.9.1 Stimulation and Injury of the Outlet Root

The stimulation and injury of the outlet root are the key points to be paid attention to and prevent in VBE lumbar fusion surgery. The main preventive measures are as follows: ① Carefully analyze the imaging data before operation, understand the anatomy and course of nerve, and eliminate the variation. ② The position of the puncture needle shall not be outside or above. ③ When the trephine is used, it shall not exceed the ventral side of the facet joint. The remaining bone blocks shall be cut off with a semi trephine or resected with laminectomy punch under direct vision to avoid trephine damage. ④ When dealing with the intervertebral space, if you see the outlet root, you can readjust the channel and block the nerve root to ensure that there is no nerve root in the operation area.

5.9.2 Injury of Exiting Root and Dural Sac

Preventive measures include: ① The position of puncture needle should not be too inward. ② When using the trephine, it shall not exceed the medial edge of the pedicle, and the remaining bone blocks shall be cut off with a semi trephine or resected with laminectomy punch to avoid trephine injury. ③ If dural sac and traversing root are seen during treatment of intervertebral space or decompression, the nerve root retractor can be used to pull it apart.

5.9.3 Injury of Vessels and Organs in Front of Vertebral

The main preventive measures are to pay great attention to the depth of the instrument during the operation. The instruments are limited in depth, and the head end and tail end are marked. Pay attention to observation under the microscope. When the instrument handle touches the channel, it means that it has entered the intervertebral space more than 40 mm, so pay special attention.

5.9.4 Malposition of Interbody Fusion Cage

The preventive measures are as follows: ① Carefully analyze the imaging data before operation and plan the operation path. ② The fusion cage should not be placed in one place at one time during implantation, but can be placed step by step, and adjusted by frontal and lateral fluoroscopy. ③ Do not loosen the handle holding of the fuser before the final confirmation of the position. If the position is not satisfactory after the cage is placed and opened, the cage can be reset and adjusted again (Figures 5.24 and 5.25).

5.9.5 Nonunion of Bone Graft

The preventive measures are as follows: ① Take autologous bone as much as possible for bone grafting. ② When autologous bone is not sufficient, allogeneic bone or artificial bone needs to be implanted. ③ Factors that promote bone formation, such as bone morphogenetic protein, can also be used.

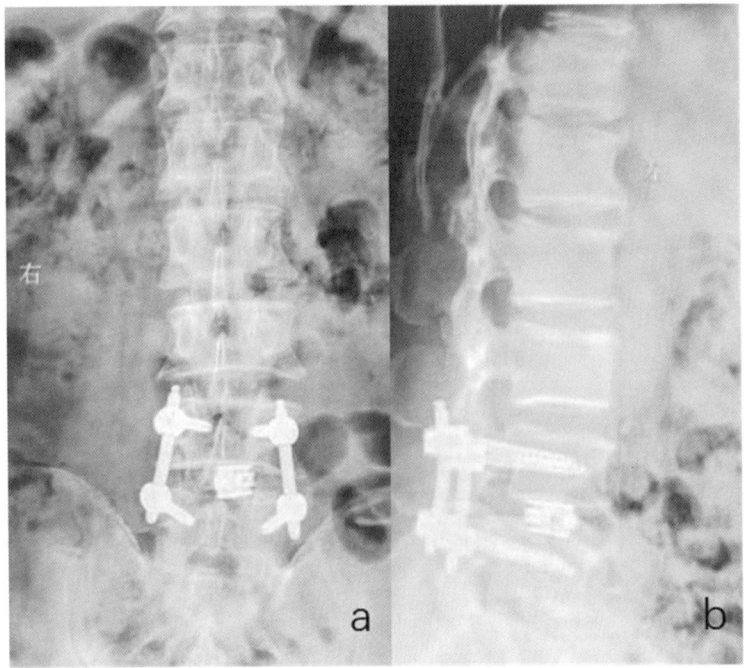

FIG. 5.24 X-ray images at 4 days after operation.
(a) Anteroposterior view; (b) lateral view.

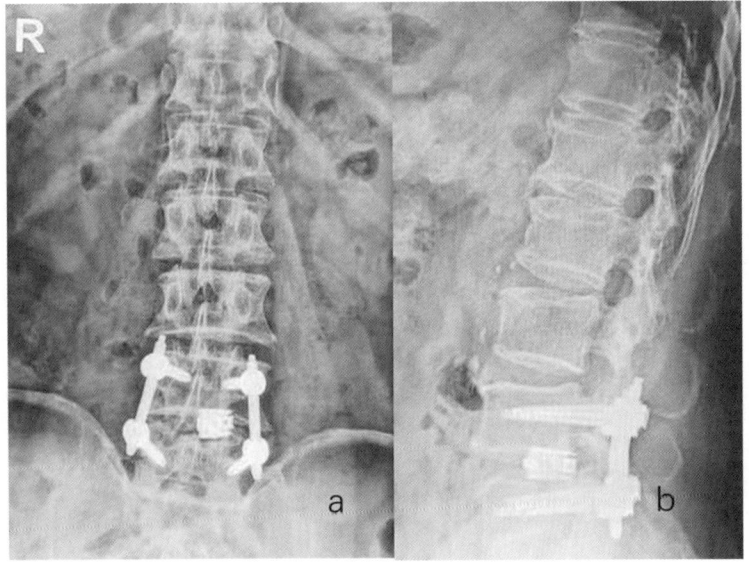

FIG. 5.25 X-ray shows malposition of cage at 3 months after operation.
(a) Anteroposterior view; (b) lateral view.

References

[1] Heemskerk J.L., Akinduro O.O., Clifton W., et al. (2021) Long-term clinical outcome of minimally invasive versus open single-level transforaminal lumbar interbody fusion for degenerative lumbar diseases: A meta-analysis, *Spine J.*

[2] Meng B., Bunch J., Burton D., et al. (2021) Lumbar interbody fusion: Recent advances in surgical techniques and bone healing strategies, *Eur. Spine J.* **30**(1), 22.

[3] Jain D., Ray W.Z., Vaccaro A.R. (2020) Advances in techniques and technology in minimally invasive lumbar interbody spinal fusion, *JBJS Rev.* **8**(4), e0171.

[4] Yao Y., Zhang H., Wu J., et al. (2017) Minimally invasive transforaminal lumbar interbody fusion versus percutaneous endoscopic lumbar discectomy: Revision surgery for recurrent herniation after microendoscopic discectomy, *World Neurosurg.* **99**, 89.

[5] Yang J.C. (2019) Current problems and challenges for percutaneous endoscopic transforaminal lumbar interbody fusio, *Zhonghua Yi Xue Za Zhi.* **99**(33), 2566.

[6] Hwa Eum J., Hwa Heo D., Son S.K., et al. (2016) Percutaneous biportal endoscopic decompression for lumbar spinal stenosis: A technical note and preliminary clinical results, *J. Neurosurg. Spine* **24**(4), 602.

[7] Heo D.H., Son S.K., Eum J.H., et al. (2017) Fully endoscopic lumbar interbody fusion using a percutaneous unilateral biportal endoscopic technique: Technical note and preliminary clinical results, *Neurosurg. Focus* **43**(2), E8.

[8] Kambin P., Sampson S. (1986) Posterolateral percutaneous suction-excision of herniated lumbar intervertebral discs. Report of interim results, *Clin. Orthop. Relat. Res.* (207), 37.

[9] Jie L., WenboDiao, Yiming L., et al. (2019) Visual trephine for foraminoplasty in percutaneous endoscopic transforaminal discectomy, *Orthop. J. China* **27**(24), 2242.

[10] Simao S., Xiaom X., Dun W., et al. (2021) Effectiveness and safety of visualized trephine used in transforaminal endoscopy, *Orthop. J. China* **29**(1), 18.

[11] Hardenbrook M., Lombardo S., Wilson M.C., et al. (2016) The anatomic rationale for transforaminal endoscopic interbody fusion: A cadaveric analysis, *Neurosurg. Focus* **40**(2), E12.

[12] Xin G., Shi-Sheng H., Hai-Long Z. (2013) Morphometric analysis of the YESS and TESSYS techniques of percutaneous transforaminal endoscopic lumbar discectomy, *Clin. Anat.* **26**(6), 728.

[13] Neidre A., MacNab I. (1983) Anomalies of the lumbosacral nerve roots. Review of 16 cases and classification, *Spine (Phila Pa 1976)* **8**(3), 294.

[14] Burke S.M., Safain M.G., Kryzanski J., et al. (2013) Nerve root anomalies: Implications for transforaminal lumbar interbody fusion surgery and a review of the Neidre and Macnab classification system, *Neurosurg. Focus* **35**(2), E9.

Chapter 6

Clinical Application of V-Shape Bichannel Endoscopy

Section Editors:

Haijian Ni, MD
Yingchuan Zhao, MD
Yunshan Fan, MD
Fangjing Chen, MD
Shunzhi Yu, MD
Kaiming Wang, MD
Peitai Liu, MD
Deshun Yang, MD
Ziquan Shen, MD

Currently, the V-shape bichannel endoscopy is mainly used for lateral transforaminal minimally invasive surgery, including transforaminal endoscopic lumbar discectomy and lumbar interbody fusion. Particularly, in cases of simple decompression, which is difficult for foraminoplasty and transforaminal intervertebral fusion, it has significant advantages due to its high efficiency, safety, and convenience.

6.1 Application of V-Shape Bichannel Endoscopy in Lumbar Decompression

Case 1
Abstract
The patient complained of recurrent low back pain and posterolateral left leg pain for more than one year. The symptoms became severe during the last month. The pain was obvious when walking, and eased after bed rest. MRI demonstrated L5/S1 intervertebral disc herniation to the left side. According to the clinical history and preoperative examination, VBE assisted discectomy *via* transforaminal approach was performed under general anesthesia.

Patient information

Medical history: A 45-year-old male, company employee, came to Shanghai Tenth People's Hospital with recurrent low back pain and posterolateral left leg pain for more than one year. The symptoms became severe during the last month. No particular previous medical history.

Physical examination: The movement of extremities was acceptable, and the physical curvature of spine existed. No deformity. Limitation of lumbar motion, intermittent claudication of the left lower limbs. The sensation of lower extremities was normal, and the muscle strength of the lower extremities was MRC grade 5. The straight leg raising test of the left lower limb was positive at 60°. The knee-jerk reflexes and Achilles's tendon reflexes of both lower limbs were (−).

Imaging examination: CT and MRI show L5/S1 para-central intervertebral disc herniation at the left side. The dural sac and nerve root were compressed.

Preoperative diagnosis: Lumbar disc herniation (L5/S1).

Case analysis

MRI demonstrated L5/S1 para-central intervertebral disc herniation at the left side (Figure 6.1). The anteroposterior lumbar radiographs showed low iliac crest but hypertrophic facet joints, and the distance between L5/S1 interlaminar space was small (Figure 6.2). The lateral radiograph showed that the ventral side of the facet joints was in close contact with the posterior edge of the vertebral body, suggesting that the anteroposterior diameter of the intervertebral foramen was small (Figure 6.2). Due to the strong willingness of the patient to receive surgery under local anesthesia, foraminoplasty would be inevitable for lateral approach (Figure 6.3). However, under the coaxial endoscope, trephine or drill is easy to slip and deviate to the ventral side, resulting in low efficiency; while the external visual trephine will remove more facet joints and even destroy the articular surface. In this case, the type I V-shape bichannel endoscopy is preferable for foraminoplasty with TESSYS endoscopic system. Through the dorsal channel, trephine, drill, or ultrasonic osteotome can be directly used in the target area (Figure 6.3). Thereby, we can improve the efficiency and accuracy of foraminoplasty and avoid excessive damage to the facet joints (Figure 6.4).

Operative key points

Based on the traditional single-port endoscopic system, normal spinal endoscope would be suitable for the type I VBE cannula. During the operation, the previous stage is the same as traditional spinal endoscope technique. The working cannula was inserted until its tip docked on the anterolateral side of the superior articular process, and then the soft tissue outside the intervertebral foramen was cleaned with a radiofrequency electrode to expose the superior articular process and the ventral disc. We can estimate the articular process that needs to be removed under the endoscope. Then the traditional working cannula can be replaced by type I VBE working cannula, High-speed drill or small trephine can be introduced into the small dorsal channel to obtain a more dorsal operation space. We can directly remove the articular process.

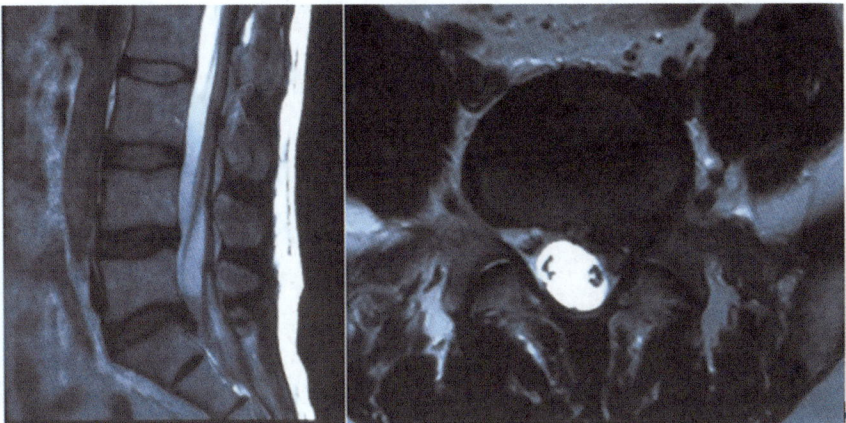

FIG. 6.1 MRI demonstrates L5/S1 para-central intervertebral disc herniation at the left side. Mid-sagittal MRI shows L5/S1 intervertebral disc herniation; cross-sectional MRI shows para-central intervertebral disc herniation at the left side.

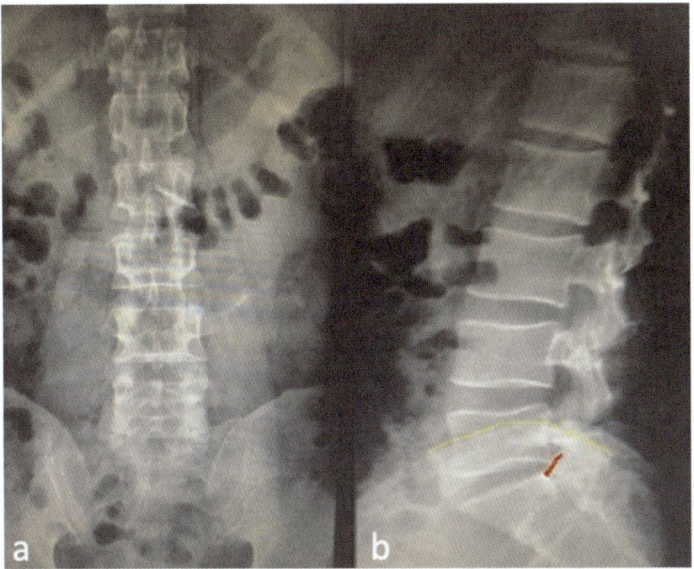

FIG. 6.2 Preoperative X-ray.
(a) The anteroposterior lumbar radiographs show the distance between L5/S1 interlaminar space was small; (b) the lateral radiograph shows that the ventral side of the facet joints are in close contact with the posterior edge of the vertebral body, suggesting that the anteroposterior diameter of the intervertebral foramen was small.

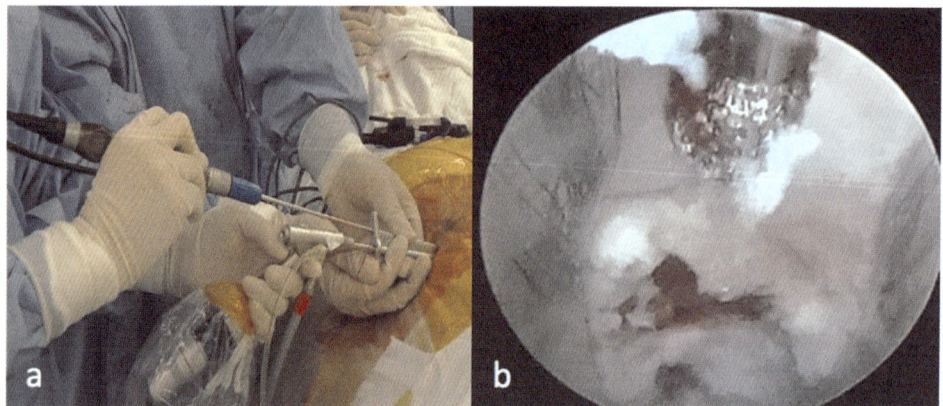

FIG. 6.3 Type I V-shape bichannel endoscopy for foraminoplasty.
(a) Intraoperative image of using high-speed bur *via* the dorsal channel of type I VBE cannula; (b) the high-speed bur could be monitored clearly under the endoscope.

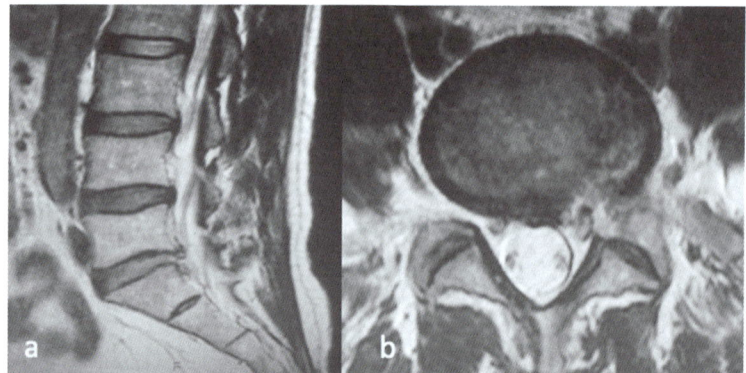

FIG. 6.4 Postoperative MRI (three days after surgery) depicted complete neural decompression and facet joint preservation.
(a) Sagittal section view; (b) cross section view.

Case 2
Abstract

This patient received posterior lumbar decompression and internal fixation (L3-S1) about 1 year ago and complained numbness and pain at the right lower extremity for about 40 days. The preoperative imaging examination showed postoperative changes in the lumbar spine, with L5/S1 intervertebral disc herniation on the right side. L5/S1 was the main responsible segment. VBE assisted lumbar discectomy *via* transforaminal approach was performed under general anesthesia for him.

Patient information

Medical history: A 59-year-old retired male who had received posterior decompression, internal fixation, and interbody fusion from L3 to S1 about 1 year ago. Symptoms such as numbness and pain reappeared in his right lower extremity for about 40 days. Previous medical history shows hypertension and cholecystectomy.

Physical examination: No deformity. The surgical incision in the lumbosacral area healed well. The lumbar motion was restricted. The straight leg raising test of the right lower limb was positive at 60°. The sensation of the posterolateral skin of the right leg was slightly decreased, and the rest of the body was roughly normal. Muscle strength of both lower limbs was MRC grade 4–5. The Achilles's tendon reflex was slightly weak. Pathological reflex (−).

Imaging examination: CT and MRI showed L5/S1 para-central intervertebral disc herniation at the left side. The dural sac and nerve root were compressed. X-ray showed postoperative changes after L3-S1 internal fixation and mild scoliosis (Figure 6.5). CT and MRI showed postoperative changes after L3-S1 internal fixation and L5/S1 intervertebral disc herniation to the right side (Figure 6.6).

Preoperative diagnosis: Lumbar disc herniation (L5/S1), post lumbar surgery status (L3-S1), post-cholecystectomy, hypertension.

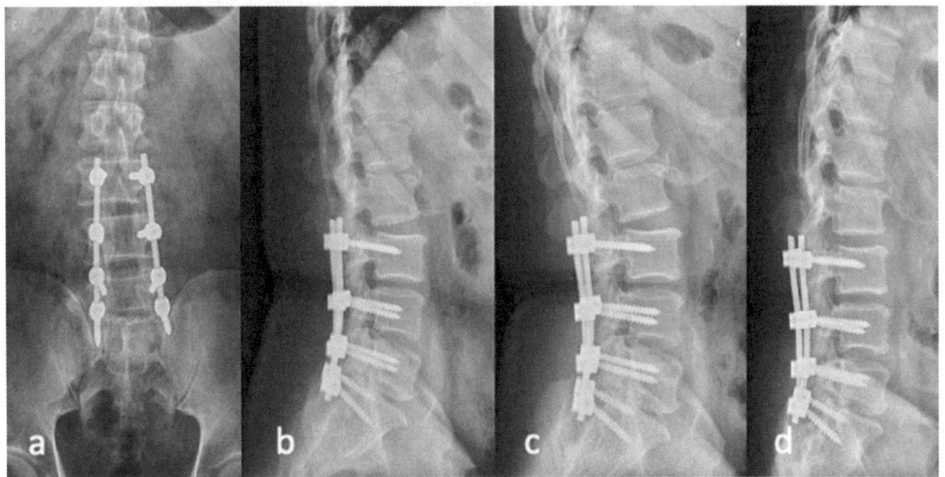

FIG. 6.5 Preoperative X-ray (anteroposterior-lateral view and dynamic view). (a),(b) Suggested that the iliac crest was high, which means that if the operation is performed from the transforaminal approach, it is difficult to insert a working channel and the operating space is limited; (c),(d) dynamic radiographs suggested L2/3 instability. Considering that the patient complained of no obvious back pain, the lumbar instability will not be dealt with at this time.

Case analysis

More than one year after the surgery, the patient complained of a recurrence of numbness and pain in the right leg, which was caused by the nerve root compression at L5/S1 level. The purpose of the operation was to remove the herniated intervertebral disc and relieve nerve compression. Because the lumbar anatomical structure was destroyed and scars were formed after the operation, it was difficult to operate *via* the posterior approach again. At the same time, due to the high iliac crest, it was difficult to insert the working channel through the transforaminal approach. The limited operating space made it difficult to perform operations such as the resection of the protruding disc tissue and decompression. In this case, the type I VBE working cannula with TESSYS endoscopic system was preferable for foraminoplasty. Through the dorsal channel of V-shape bichannel endoscopy, the high-speed bur could be directly used to perform foraminoplasty. It could enlarge the operating space effectively and quickly, which significantly improved efficiency. Therefore, we could completely remove the herniated disc mass and relieve compressed nerve roots.

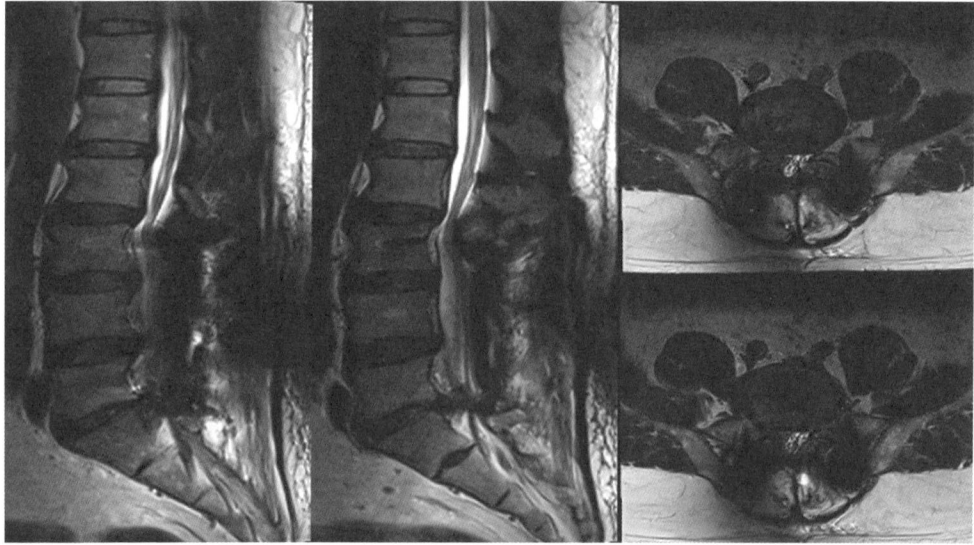

FIG. 6.6 Preoperative MRI shows postoperative changes after L3-S1 internal fixation and L5/S1 intervertebral disc herniation to the right side.

Operative key points

We could identify the target point on anteroposterior and lateral x-ray. Subsequently, the sequential dilators were introduced through the soft tissue and traditional working cannula was inserted onto the ventral portion of the ipsilateral superior facet. The radiofrequency electrode and pulposus forceps were used under the endoscope to clean the soft tissues, and the trephine was used for preliminary foraminoplasty. We then replaced the working cannula with type I VBE working cannula. Through the dorsal small channel, the high-speed bur enlarged the intervertebral foramen and the pulposus forceps exposed the structure of the spinal canal. Then, we could completely remove the disk herniation and relieve the compressed nerve roots (Figure 6.7).

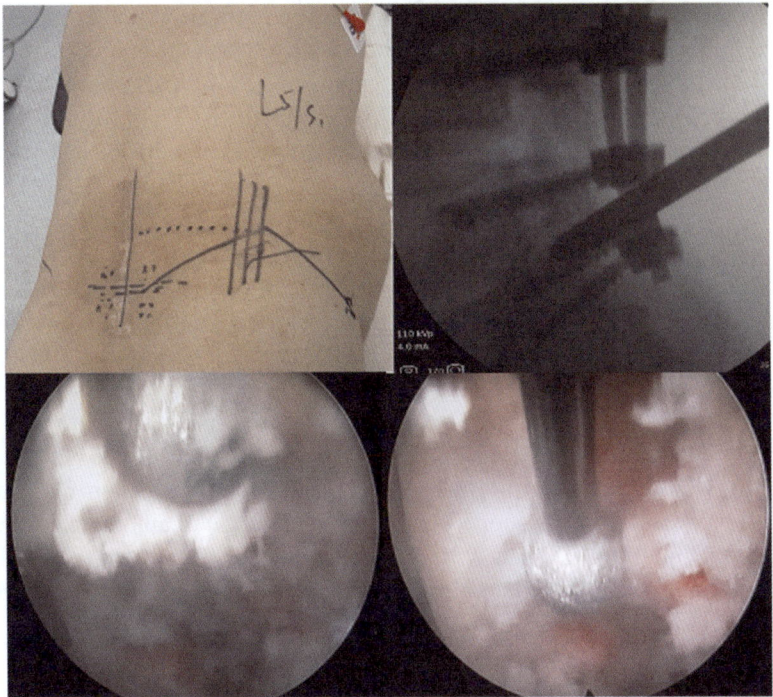

FIG. 6.7 Type I VBE working cannula for foraminoplasty. The high-speed drill enlarges the intervertebral foramen through the dorsal small channel.

6.2 Application of V-Shape Bichannel Endoscopy in Lumbar Fusion

Based on the V-shape bichannel endoscopy, VBE lumbar fusion technology is a new endoscopic lumbar fusion technology. Like MIS-TLIF, part of the articular process is removed during the operation, and the intervertebral disc can be reached directly through Kambin's triangle. The surgical path is direct and rapid, and the possibility of damage to the dural sac and nerve roots is relatively low. Moreover, the entire operation is performed under VBE endoscopic monitoring without many repeated fluoroscopies, so the operation is safe and simple. Main surgical indications include lateral lumbar spinal stenosis, lumbar spondylolisthesis, lumbar instability, and recurrent lumbar disc herniation which needs lumbar fusion.

6.2.1 VBE Lumbar Fusion for Lumbar Spinal Stenosis

Case 3
Abstract
The patient complained of low back pain for about 3 years, and hip soreness (heavier on the right side) after walking about 300 m, which could be relieved after rest.

Symptoms worsened six months ago, and the patient demonstrated antalgic gait after 100 m. After conservative treatment for 3 months, there was no significant improvement in subjective symptoms. Preoperative MRI demonstrated L4/5 paracentral intervertebral disc herniation at the right side and lateral recess stenosis. Therefore, VBE assisted decompression, bone graft fusion, and internal fixation were performed under general anesthesia.

Patient information

Medical history: A 55-year-old male, worker, complained of low back and right lower limb pain for 3 years, worsening for half a year, and intermittent claudication. No particular previous medical history.

Physical examination: Antalgic gait. No deformity. Physical curvature existed. Limitation of lumbar motion with provocative pain. Muscle strength of the right extensor hallucis muscle was MRC grade 3–4. Hypesthesia at the posterolateral skin of the right lower limb. The straight leg raising test of the right leg was positive at 60°. The knee jerk and Achilles's tendon reflexes were normal. Pathological reflex (−).

Imaging examination: CT and MRI showed L4/5 para-central intervertebral disc herniation at the right side and lateral recess stenosis. The nerve root was compressed (Figures 6.8–6.11).

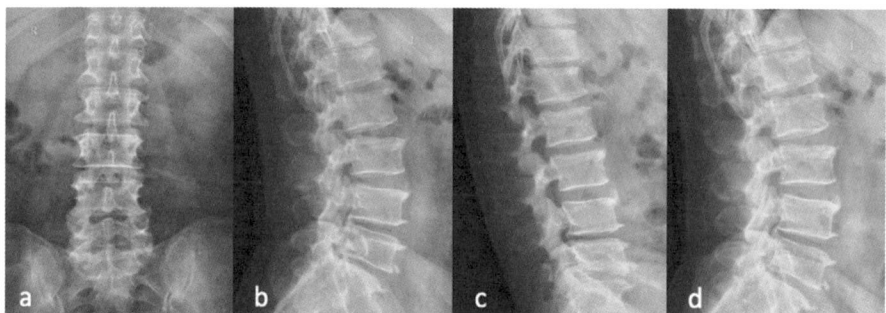

FIG. 6.8 Preoperative X-ray images.
(a), (b) X-ray shows lumbar degeneration, narrowing of the intervertebral space at L4/5, L5/S1 segments, and hyperosteogeny of facet joints; (c), (d) X-ray in dynamic position indicated mild instability of L3/4.

Preoperative diagnosis: Lumbar spinal stenosis (L4/5), lumbar disc herniation (L4/5).

Case analysis

This patient was diagnosed with L4/5 spinal stenosis and disc herniation. Considering his age and the degree of disc degeneration, and the onset of intermittent claudication appeared at the early stage, the long-term effect of endoscopic decompression was unclear. In addition, the patient's demand was minimally invasive surgical treatment. In this case, the VBE endoscopic decompression, bone graft fusion, and internal fixation is appropriate for the patient. It could minimize the surgical trauma and ensure the long-term effect.

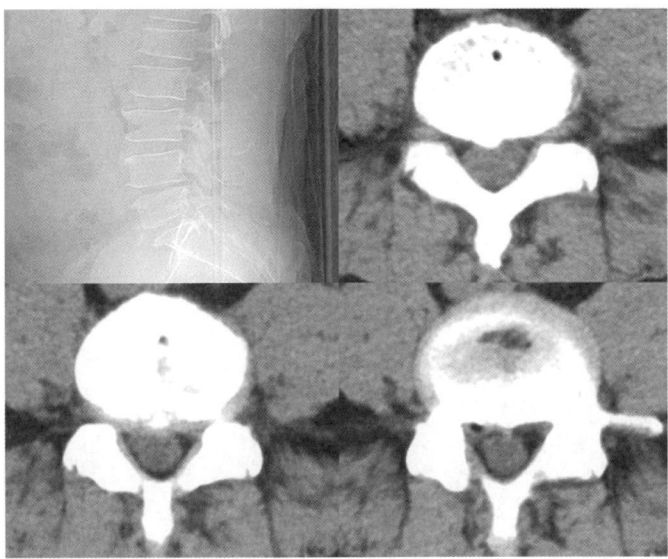

FIG. 6.9 CT of the lumbar spine shows L4/5 intervertebral disc herniation (para-central intervertebral disc herniation at the left side with calcification), facet joint hyperosteogeny, and bilateral lateral recess stenosis.

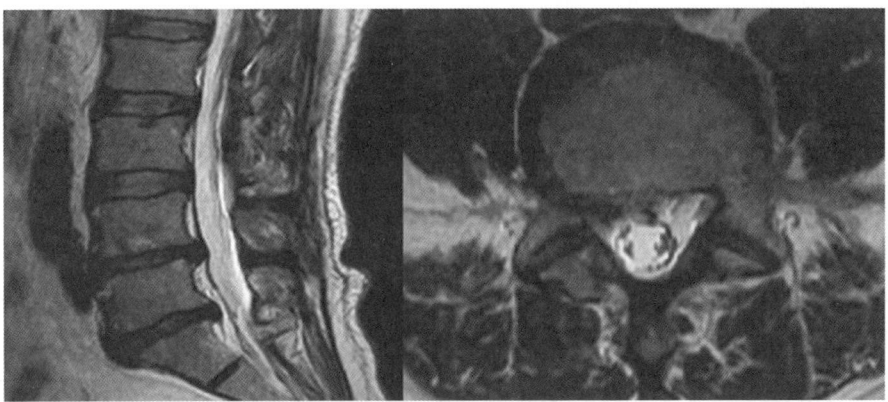

FIG. 6.10 MRI demonstrates L4/5 para-central intervertebral disc herniation at the right side and lateral recess stenosis.

Operative key points

For patients with lateral stenosis, the anatomical factors leading to the stenosis need to be analyzed. In this case, the stenosis was mainly caused by hyperosteogeny of the superior articular process and lateral intervertebral disc herniation. Therefore, using a trephine to remove part of the superior articular process, and removing the ventral intervertebral disc could achieve the purpose of decompression. The central spinal canal, nerve roots, and dural sac might not be necessary to be exposed because the partial facetectomy was relatively to the outside. Therefore, the interbody fusion could be performed before the decompression. Since the risk of dural sac and nerve root injury was low, and the nerve retraction was unnecessary, it made the surgery safer. After the fusion procedure, decompression and discectomy could be performed. The lamina and ligamentum flavum could be removed as needed. Then, the nerve root and dural sac could be examined, and the ventral intervertebral disc was removed (Figure 6.12).

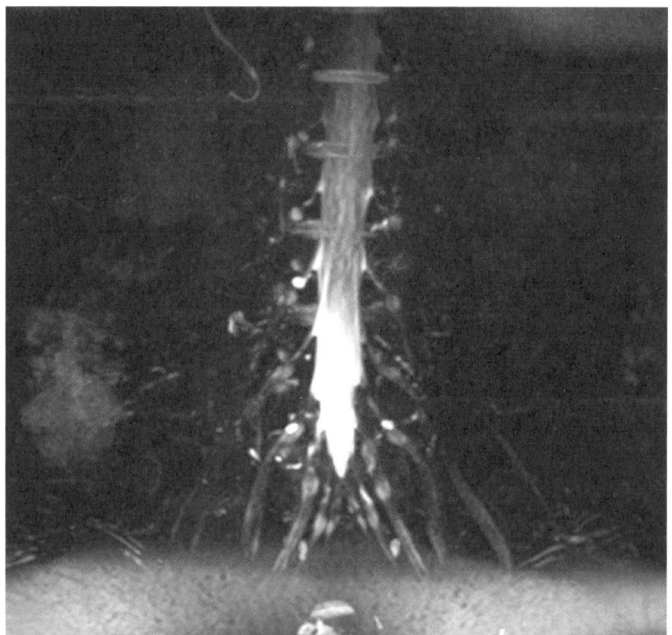

FIG. 6.11 Preoperative MRN image shows no nerve root anomaly.

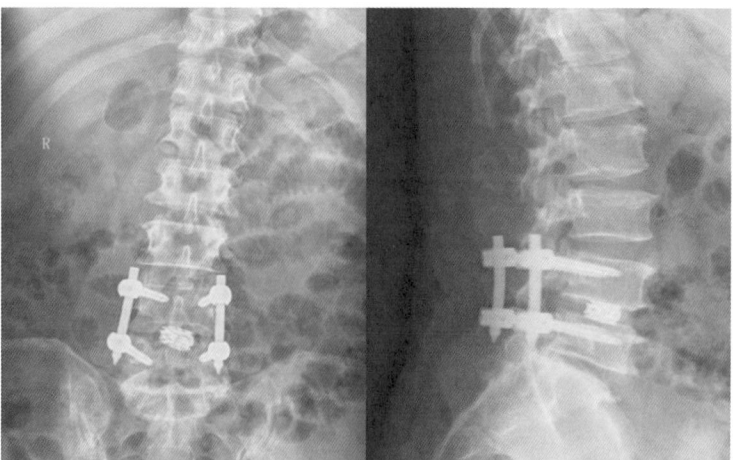

FIG. 6.12 X-ray (3 days after the operation) shows the screw-rod and the fusion cage was in a good position.

Case 4

Abstract

The patient complained of recurring low back pain for more than 3 months, and the pain had worsened in the past month with numbness and pain in the right lower extremity. The symptoms were obvious after walking and partly relieved after rest. Preoperative MRI revealed that L4/5 intervertebral disc herniation to the right side and lumbar spinal stenosis. Therefore, VBE endoscopic decompression, bone graft fusion, and internal fixation were performed under general anesthesia.

Patient information

Medical history: A 67-year-old male retired patient complained of low back pain for 3 months with aggravated pain and numbness of the right lower limb for 1 month. Diabetes was diagnosed one year ago.

Physical examination: No deformity. Limitation of lumbar motion. Hypesthesia in the right crus and foot. The rest sensation of the body was roughly normal. Muscle strength of the right extensor hallucis muscle was MRC grade 4 and the rest muscles were MRC grade 5. The straight leg raising test of the right lower limb was positive at 50°. The knee jerk and Achilles's tendon reflexes were normal. Pathological reflex (−).

Imaging examination: CT and MRI showed right extraforaminal disc at L4/5 with foraminal stenosis, and the right nerve root was compressed (Figures 6.13–6.16).

Preoperative diagnosis: Lumbar spinal stenosis (L4/5), lumbar disc herniation (L4/5), diabetes.

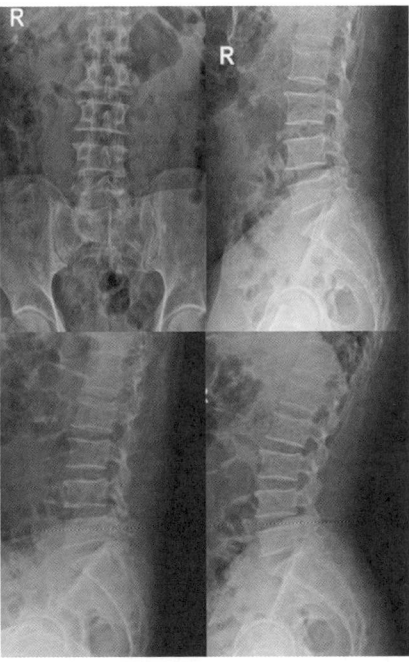

FIG. 6.13 X-ray shows lumbar degeneration, narrowing L4/5 intervertebral space, and no obvious instability or spondylolisthesis in the dynamic position.

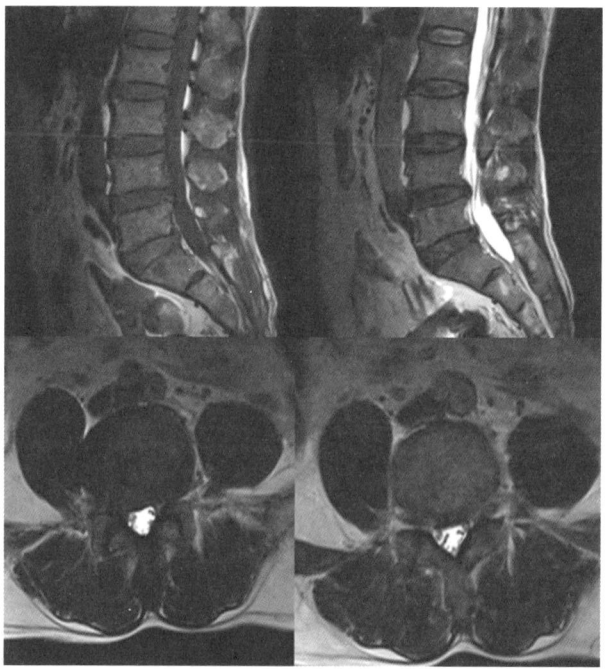

FIG. 6.14 MRI demonstrates L4/5 para-central intervertebral disc herniation at the right side and right nerve root compressing the right nerve.

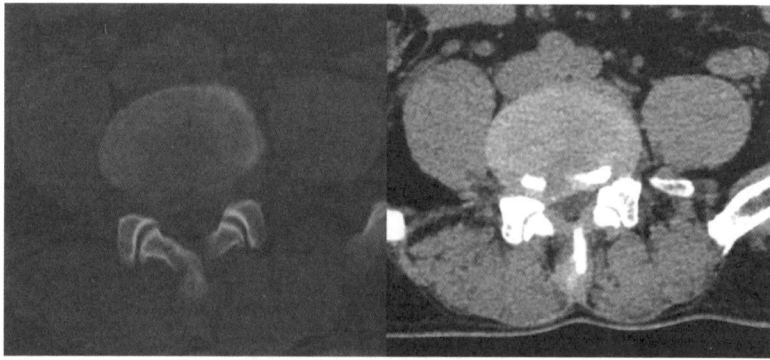

FIG. 6.15 CT of the lumbar spine shows L4/5 intervertebral disc herniation, hyperosteogeny of the facet joints, and right intervertebral foramen stenosis.

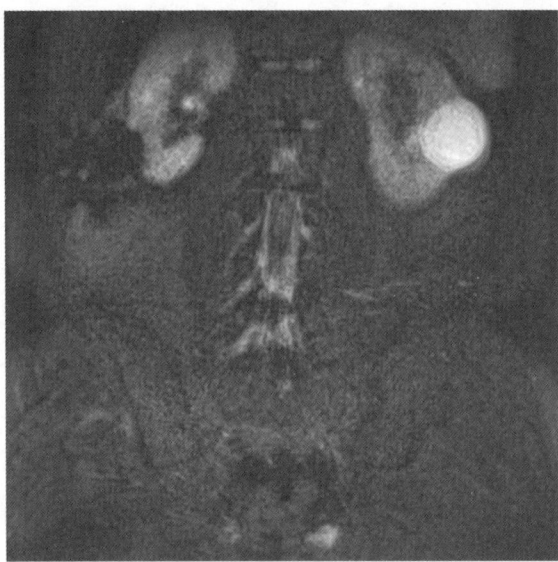

FIG. 6.16 Preoperative MRN image shows no nerve root anomaly.

Case analysis

This patient was diagnosed with L4/5 spinal stenosis and disc protrusion. The imaging examination showed that obvious hyperosteogeny of the right facet joints combined with the herniated intervertebral disc led to the lateral spinal stenosis and corresponding symptoms. Endoscopic decompression should be helpful for him. Considering the patient's age and requirements, VBE endoscopic decompression, bone graft fusion, and internal fixation were more suitable. Lumbar spinal stenosis, which is mainly stenosis on one side, was a good indication for VBE lumbar fusion.

Operative key points

The width and direction of the facet joints and lumbosacral transitional vertebra are very important for operative pathway planning. The distance from lateral to the midline and direction of trephine insertion was crucial. If the distance was too large, the trephine would head to the ventral side, which may damage the inner dural sac and nerve roots. On the contrary, if the trephine headed to the dorsal side, the facet joint resection would be insufficient and increase the risk of exiting nerve root injury. Therefore, X-ray was necessary during partial facetectomy. The inner side of the trephine should not exceed the inner pedicle edge in the anterior view, and the outer side does not exceed the front edge of the articular process joints in the lateral view. In this position, even if the bone mass was not completely disconnected or removed, we could replace the trephine with a half-thread trephine, arc osteotome, pulposus forceps, straight forceps, and other tools under endoscopy to remove the bone mass and avoid nerve injuries (Figure 6.17).

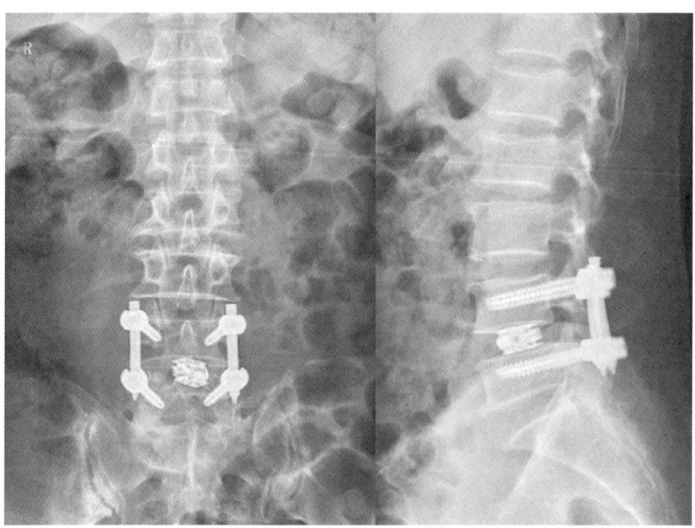

FIG. 6.17 X-ray after the operation shows the screw-rod and the fusion cage was in a good position.

Case 5

Abstract

The patient complained of lower back pain for more than 10 years, pain in both lower limbs (mainly in the lateral lower leg), and numbness (mainly in the left foot) for one year. The symptoms relieved after rest. Pain and numbness were aggravated in the past month. Preoperative MRI revealed lumbar spinal stenosis (L4/5) and mild spondylolisthesis (I°, L4). After evaluation, VBE endoscopic decompression, bone graft fusion, and internal fixation were performed under general anesthesia.

Patient information

Medical history: A 71-year-old retired man complained of low back pain for more than 10 years and pain and numbness in both lower limbs for one year. The symptoms aggravated over the last month. Previous history of atrial premature beats.

Physical examination: Lumbar curvature existed. Lumbar spinous process tenderness and percussion tenderness (+). The straight leg raising test of the left lower limb was positive at 60°. Hypesthesiain at both lower extremities. Muscle strength of both lower limbs: iliopsoas muscle and quadriceps were MRC grade 4; tibialis anterior and extensor hallucis muscle were MRC grade 4 (left) and grade 5 (right). Weakened knee jerk and Achilles's tendon reflexes. Pathological reflex (−).

Imaging examination: CT and MRI showed lumbar spinal stenosis (L4/5) and mild spondylolisthesis (I°, L4). MRN image showed no nerve root anomaly (Figures 6.18–6.21).

Preoperative diagnosis: Lumbar spinal stenosis (L4/5), lumbar spondylolisthesis (I°, L4), atrial premature beats.

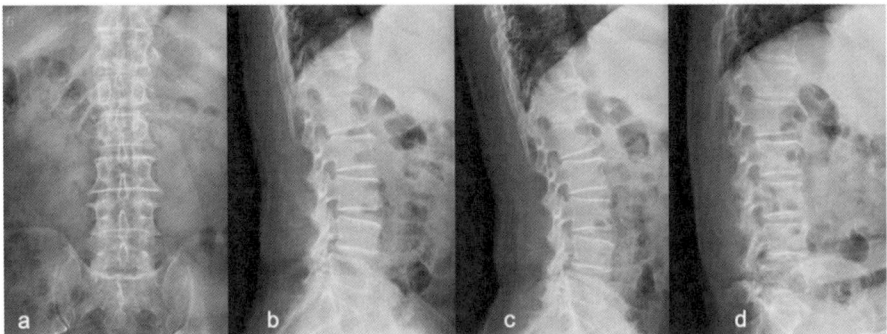

FIG. 6.18　Preoperative X-ray.
(a), (b) Radiographs show L4 spondylolisthesis (I°); (c), (d) the dynamic position indicated mild instability of L4.

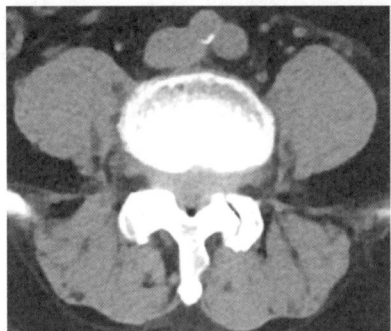

FIG. 6.19　Preoperative CT images in transverse section showed bilateral nerve compression.

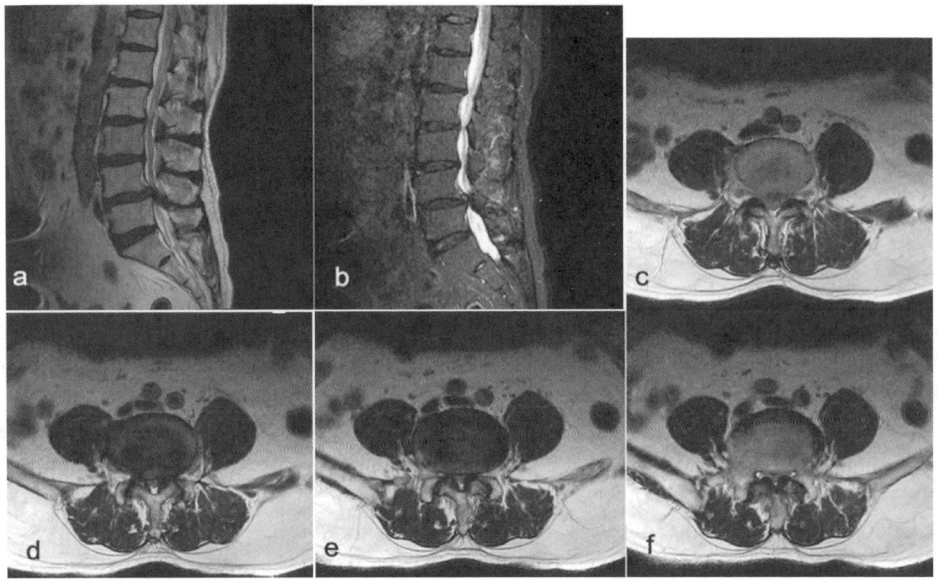

FIG. 6.20　Preoperative MRI demonstrates L4 spondylolisthesis with spinal stenosis.
(a), (b) Sagittal section view; (c)–(f) cross section view.

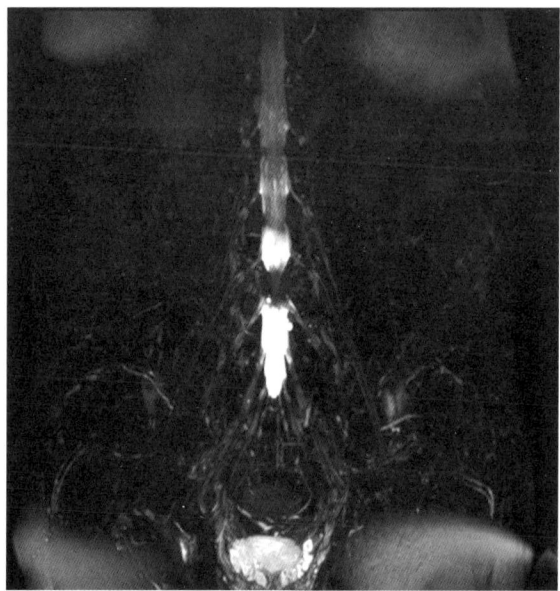

FIG. 6.21   MRN image shows no nerve root anomaly.

Case analysis

The main cause of symptoms is spinal stenosis, which was mainly due to mild spondylolisthesis of the upper vertebral body, disc herniation, and compression of the inferior articular process on both sides. Due to the symptoms of bilateral claudication and the imaging examination revealing bilateral stenosis, bilateral decompression was necessary. For such cases, VBE lumbar decompression and fusion can be performed from one side, and the other side can be decompressed by trephine with a traditional single-port endoscopic system. Thus, we can perform bilateral decompression and intervertebral fusion at the same time.

Operative key points

Because the upper large channel of VBE working cannula and the large-diameter trephine used during partial facetectomy are circular, the residual base after the partial facetectomy is also arc-shaped. Therefore, it is necessary to use laminectomy punch to further decompress the lateral recess to ensure complete decompression. For bilateral lateral stenosis, unilateral approach with bilateral decompression might increase unnecessary dorsal dural sac exposure. In addition, it would increase the irritation of postoperative hemorrhage to the dural sac and the occurrence of dural sac adhesion. Therefore, a traditional single-port endoscopic system was recommended for decompression on the other side. According to this strategy, VBE decompression and interbody fusion were performed on one side, and a traditional endoscopic system was used for decompression on the other side. The two endoscopic systems would not interfere with each other, and the two operations could be separately performed by two surgeons at the same time. Therefore, compared with unilateral VBE decompression and fusion, it would not significantly increase the operation time, this strategy could also be one of the advantages of the VBE system (Figures 6.22–6.24).

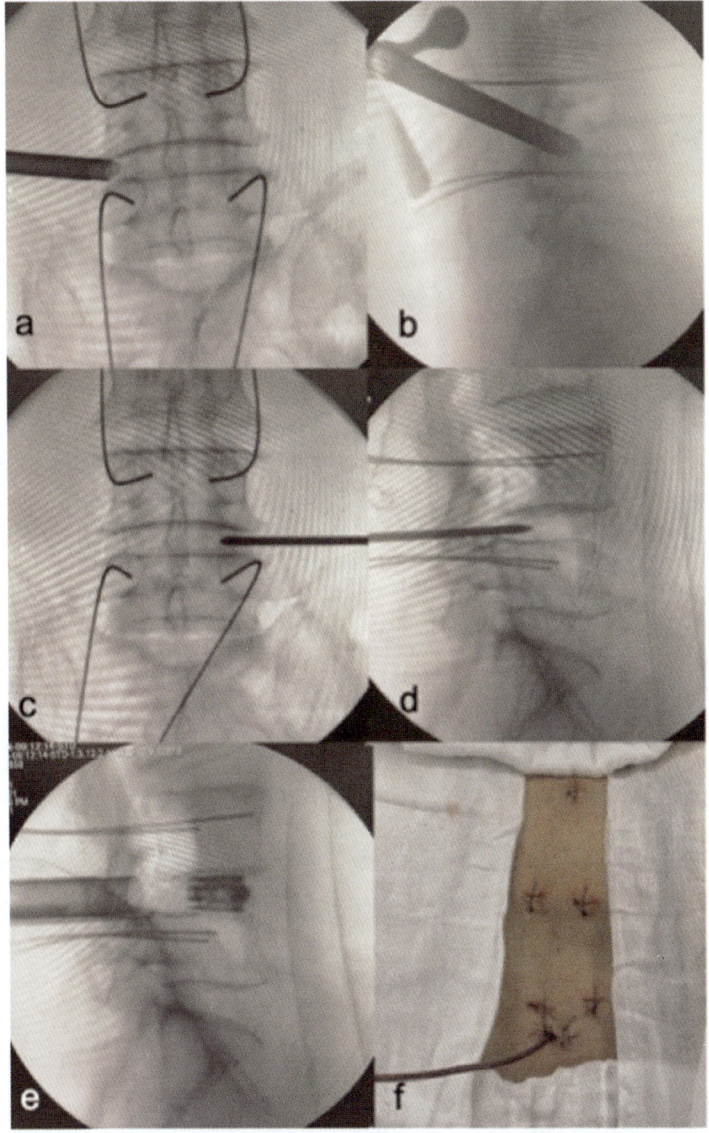

FIG. 6.22 Images of intraoperative operation.
(a), (b) Decompression was performed at one side with traditional technique; (c), (d) puncture was performed at the other side with VBE technique; (e) decompression and fusion was performed; (f) the appearance of the postoperative incision.

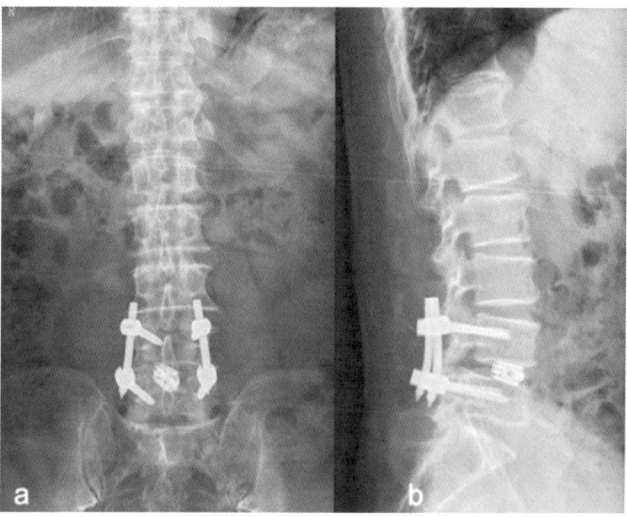

FIG. 6.23 X-ray (3 days after the operation) shows the internal fixation and the fusion cage were in good position.

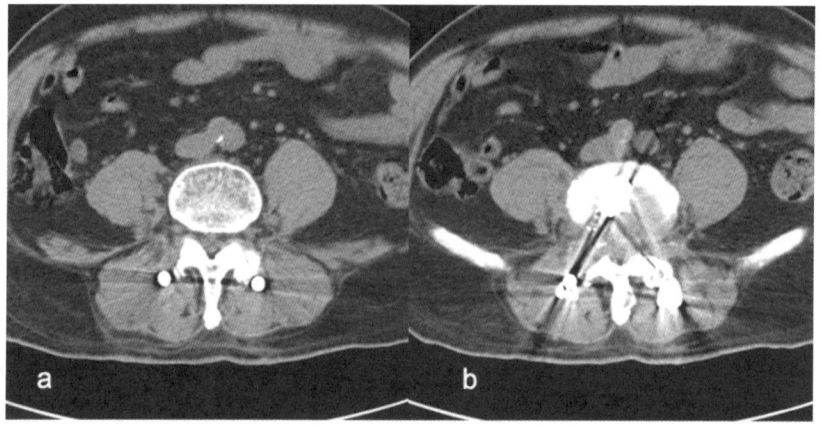

FIG. 6.24 CT images (3 days after the operation) in transverse section.
(a),(b) Different level of cross section view.

Case 6
Abstract

The patient complained back pain for 5 years, but had no significant improvement with conservative treatment. Symptoms were significantly aggravated in the past six months, and pain in the waist and hips appeared unbearable after walking for more than ten minutes. The symptoms relieved after resting. Imaging examination showed L3/4, L4/5 spinal stenosis, and L4 spondylolisthesis. Therefore, VBE endoscopic decompression, bone graft fusion, and internal fixation were performed under general anesthesia.

Patient information

Medical history: A 73-year-old retired woman complained of repeated low back pain for 5 years, and hip pain which began one half years ago.

Physical examination: Lumbar curvature existed. Lumbar spinous process tenderness (+), and percussion tenderness (−). The straight leg raising test for both lower limbs was negative. Muscle strength of both lower limbs: iliopsoas muscle, quadriceps, and tibialis anterior were MRC grade 4; gastrocnemius and extensor hallucis muscle were MRC grade 5. Weakened knee jerk and Achilles's tendon reflexes. Pathological reflex (−).

Imaging examination: X-ray, CT and MRI show lumbar spinal stenosis (L3/4, L4/5) and L4 spondylolisthesis (Figures 6.25–6.27).

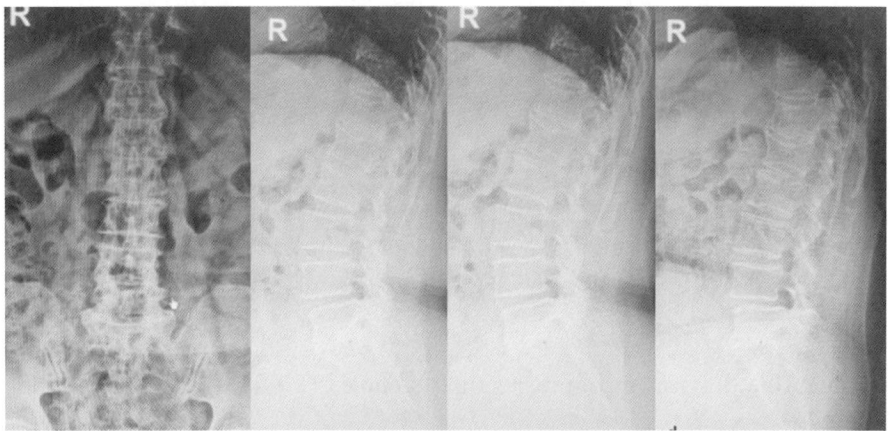

FIG. 6.25 L3/4 and L4/5 articular process hyperosteogeny and L4 spondylolisthesis.

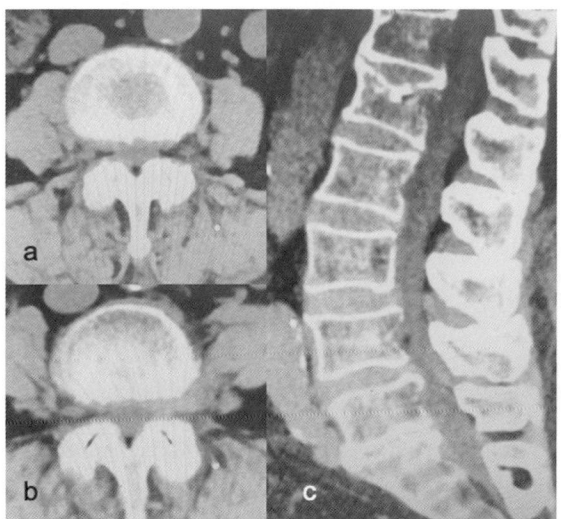

FIG. 6.26 Preoperative CT image shows L3/4 and L4/5 spinal stenosis.
(a),(b) Cross section view; (c) sagittal section view.

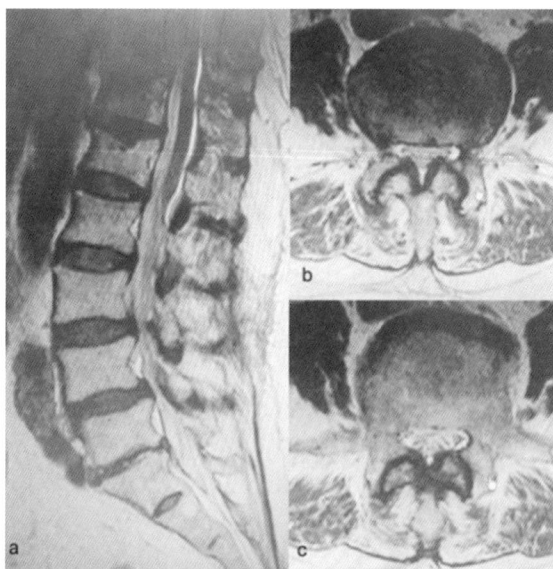

FIG. 6.27 MRI shows L3/4 and L4/5 articular process hyperosteogeny, ligamentum flavum hypertrophy, spinal stenosis, and L4 spondylolisthesis.

(a) Sagittal section view; (b),(c) cross section view.

Preoperative diagnosis: Lumbar spinal stenosis (L3/4, L4/5), lumbar spondylolisthesis (L4).

Case analysis

The L3/4 and L4/5 spinal stenosis were mainly caused by the pathological development of the inferior articular process. The vertebra tended to slide forward, resulting in relative spinal stenosis. Especially in the situation of spinal movement and weight bearing status, the stenosis might be aggravated. Therefore, the key consideration for such patients was to relieve the compression of the inferior articular process during the surgery. On the one hand, removal of the inferior articular process would reduce the compression, and on the other hand, indirect decompression could be achieved through the expansion of the intervertebral space and bone graft fusion.

Operative key points

Just like MIS-TLIF, only one incision was needed for two adjacent level lumbar fusion with the VBE system. The VBE working cannula could be adjusted to the cephalic or caudal side to visualize the two adjacent levels. The articular processes of these two levels could be exposed and partial resected following the anatomical structure. The fusion and decompression could be completed. The VBE system showed high efficiency and minimal trauma in performing two adjacent level lumbar fusion surgery, and its operation time was not longer than that of MIS-TLIF (Figures 6.28–6.33).

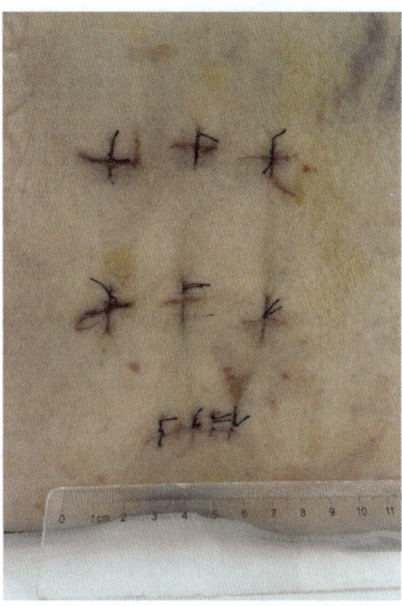

FIG. 6.28 Surgical incision. Only one incision was needed. The direction of the VBE working cannula could be adjusted to the cephalic or caudal side to visualize the two adjacent levels.

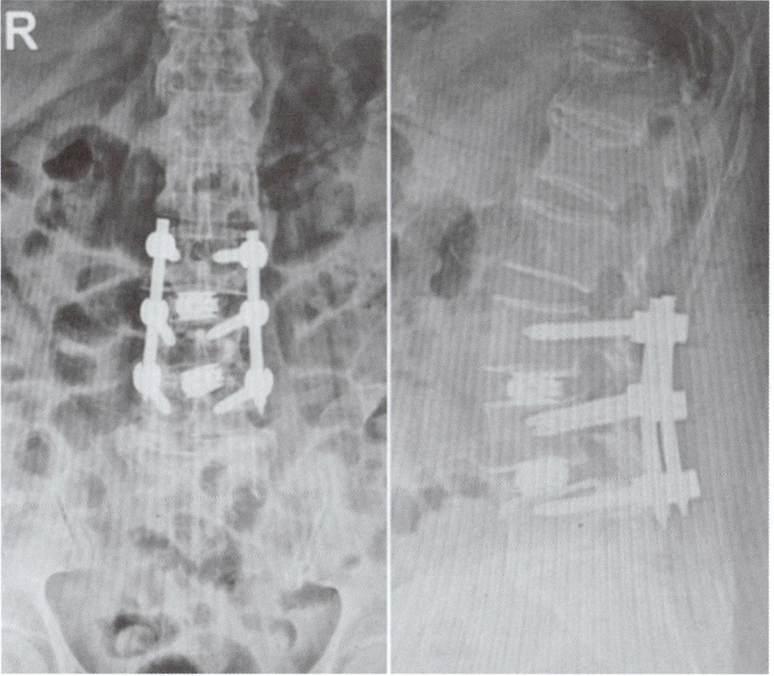

FIG. 6.29 X-ray on postoperative day 4 shows the internal fixation and the fusion cage were in a good position.

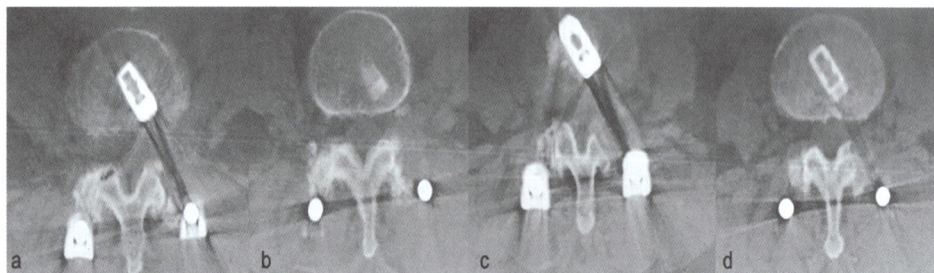

FIG. 6.30 CT on postoperative day 4 of transverse section shows the internal fixation and the decompression of neural elements were satisfactory.
(a),(b) Cross section view of L3/4; (c), (d) cross section view of L4/5.

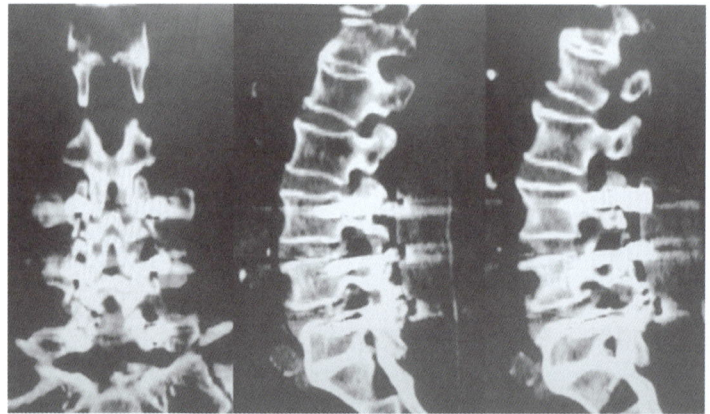

FIG. 6.31 CT image in coronal section view and sagittal section view.

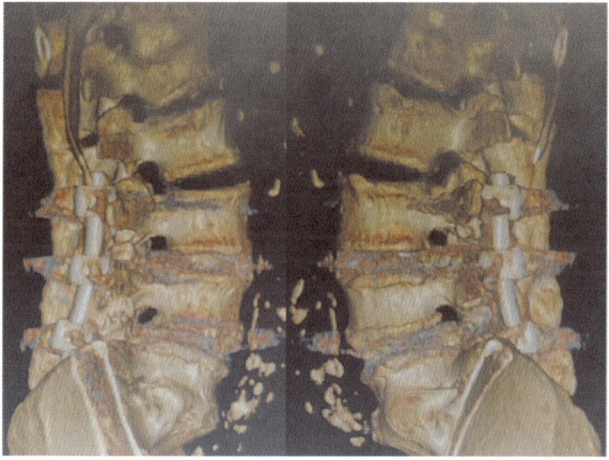

FIG. 6.32 CT three-dimensional reconstruction images showing L4 correction with restoration of the physiological curvature of the lumbar.

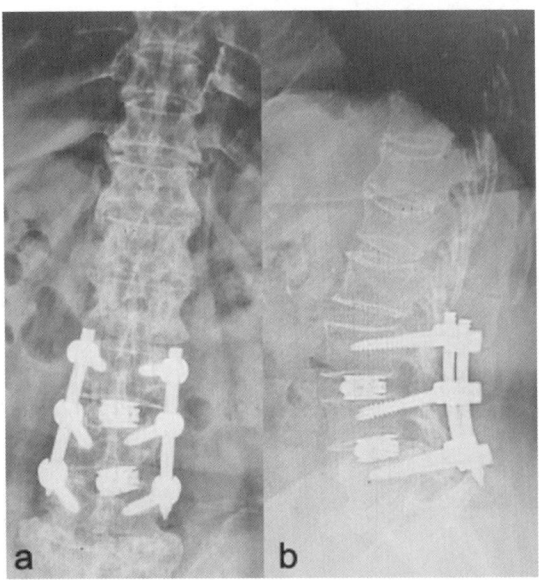

FIG. 6.33 X-ray images at 3 months after surgery shows that the internal fixation position was good.

(a) Anteroposterior view; (b) lateral view.

6.2.2 VBE Lumbar Fusion for Spondylolisthesis

Case 7

Abstract

The patient complained of low back pain and numbness in both lower limbs for more than one year, which was obvious during standing or walking. Symptoms could not be relieved by conservative treatment and were gradually aggravated. The X-ray, CT, and MRI revealed lumbar spondylolisthesis (I°, L4). Therefore, VBE endoscopic decompression, bone graft fusion, and internal fixation were performed under general anesthesia.

Patient information

Medical history: A 73-year-old retired woman complained of low back pain and numbness in both lower limbs for more than one year. Past medical history of systemic lupus erythematosus. Medication history of prednisolone acetate.

Physical examination: Mild thoracic kyphosis. Lumbar curvature existed. Lumbar tenderness and percussion tenderness (+). Limitation of lumbar motion. Hypesthesiain of both lower extremities. Muscle strength of extensor hallucis muscle was MRC grade 3 (left) and grade 4 (right). The straight leg raising test for both lower limbs was negative. Weakened knee jerk and Achilles's tendon reflexes. Pathological reflex (−).

Imaging examination: X-ray, CT, and MRI showed L4 spondylolisthesis, proliferation and cohesion of articular process, hyperplasia, and hypertrophy of the ligamentum flavum, and spinal stenosis (Figures 6.34–6.37).

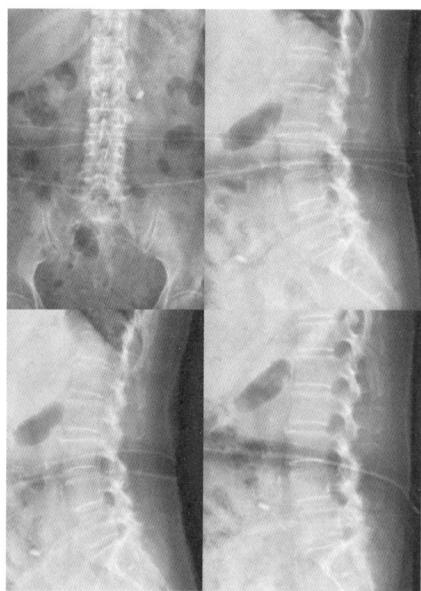
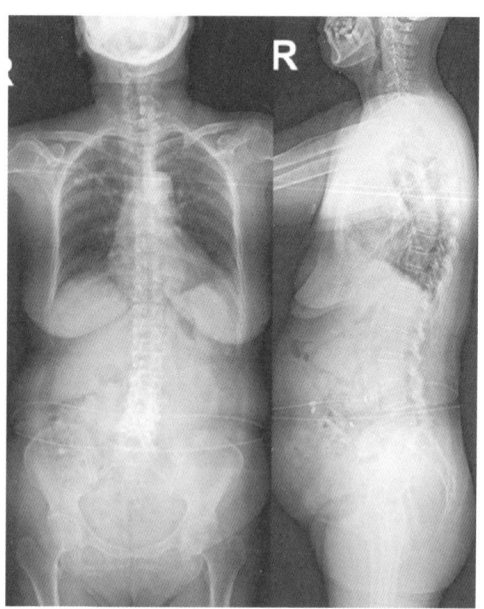

FIG. 6.34 Preoperative X-ray shows L4 spondylolisthesis (I°) and osteoporosis.

FIG. 6.35 Standing anteroposterior and lateral view of full spine shows degenerative scoliosis and L4 spondylolisthesis (I°).

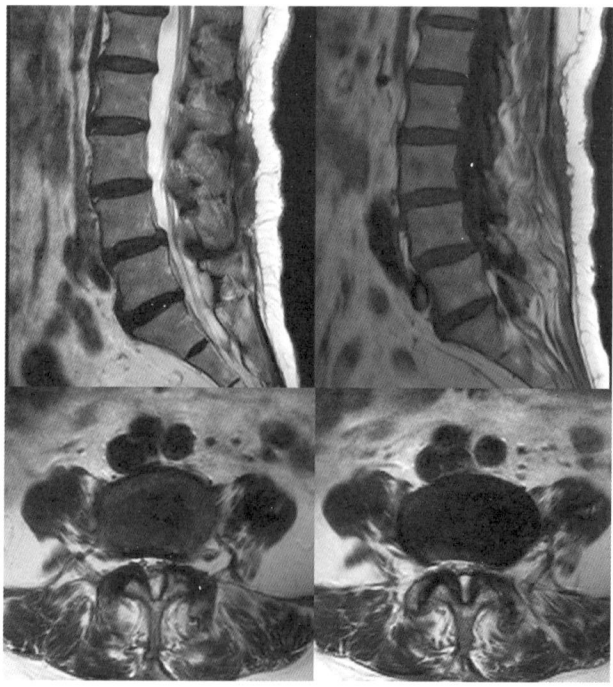

FIG. 6.36 MRI demonstrates L4 spondylolisthesis, articular process hyperosteogeny, and ligamentum flavum hypertrophy.

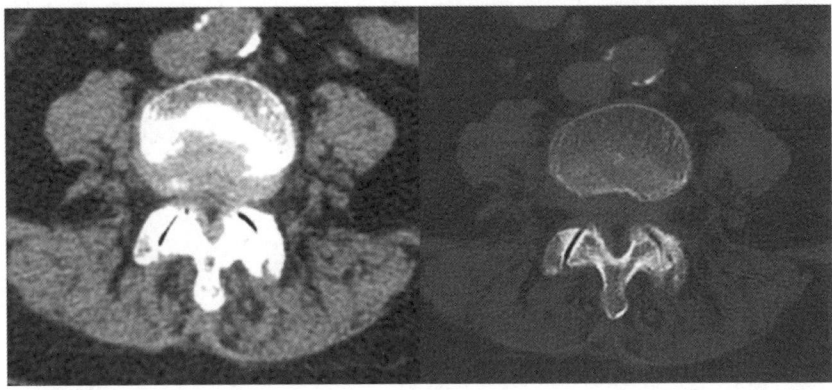

FIG. 6.37 CT of the lumbar spine shows L4/5 spinal stenosis and L4 spondylolisthesis.

Preoperative diagnosis: Lumbar spondylolisthesis (I°, L4), osteoporosis, systemic lupus erythematosus.

Case analysis

The patient complained of persistent low back pain with numbness in both lower extremities. According to physical and imaging examinations, L4 spondylolisthesis combined with facet joint hyperosteogeny and ligamentum flavum hypertrophy leaded to L4/5 spinal stenosis. The main symptoms caused by lumbar spondylolisthesis included segmental instability and degenerative changes secondary to spondylolisthesis. The main cause of the symptoms needed to be carefully analyzed. If spondylolisthesis was the main reason, reduction, fixation, and fusion can relieve the symptoms; if there were physical pressuring substance such as joint hyperosteogeny, ligamentum flavum hyperplasia, and intervertebral disc herniation, further decompression would be required. The surgeon must carefully inquire about the medical history in detail, carry out physical examination and analyze the imaging examination comprehensively before the operation.

Operative key points

For this patient with osteoporosis, attention should be paid to accurate positioning during percutaneous screw placement to avoid repeated adjustments leading to postoperative screw migration. At the same time, pedicle screws with cement augmentation can also be used. In the process of handling the intervertebral space, the surgeon needed to protect the endplate to avoid endplate bone damage, which might result in collapse and displacement of the fusion cage. For patients with a low degree of spondylolisthesis, the reduction could be completed by adjusting the expandable fusion cage and internal fixation (Figure 6.38).

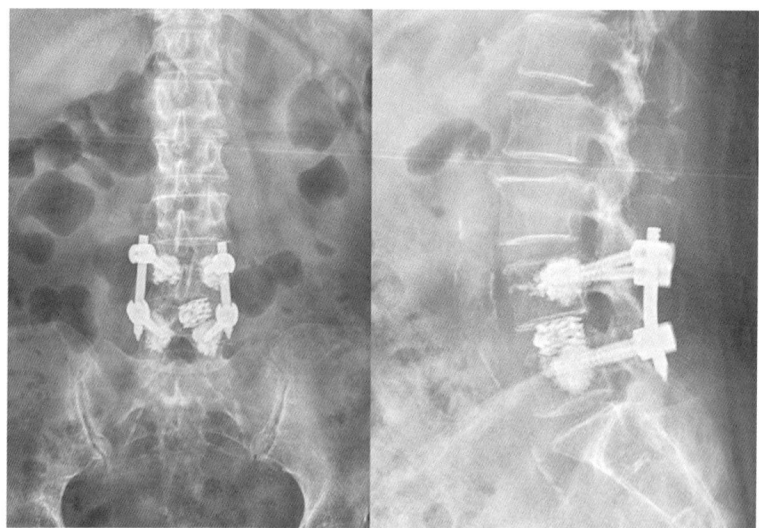

FIG. 6.38 X-rays in anteroposterior-lateral position. Due to osteoporosis, pedicle screws with cement augmentation were used.

Case 8
Abstract

The patient complained of lumbosacral pain and numbness of both lower extremities for one year, worsening in the last three months. Imaging examination revealed L5 spondylolisthesis (I°) and lumbar spinal stenosis. After evaluation, VBE assisted decompression, bone graft fusion, and internal fixation were performed under general anesthesia.

Patient information

Medical history: A 59-year-old male worker complained of lumbosacral pain and numbness of both lower extremities for one year, aggravated for the last three months. No particular previous medical history.

Physical examination: Physical curvature existed. Mild pain in the lumbosacral area. Pain and numbness on the outer thigh, crus, back of the foot, and sole of both lower limbs, especially the right lower limb. The straight leg raising test of the left lower limb was positive at 60°, and the augment test was positive. The straight leg raising test of the right lower limb was positive at 30°. Muscle strength of iliopsoas muscle was MRC grade 5 (left) and grade 4 (right). The knee jerk and Achilles's tendon reflexes are normal. Pathological reflex (−). The VAS score for low back pain was 7 points, and the right lower limb was 4 points.

Imaging examination: X-ray revealed L5 spondylolisthesis (I°) (Figure 6.39). CT and MRI showed L5 spondylolisthesis (I°), lumbar spinal canal stenosis, and lumbar disc herniation (L5/S1).

Preoperative diagnosis: Lumbar spondylolisthesis (L5/I°), lumbar spinal stenosis, lumbar disc herniation (L5/S1).

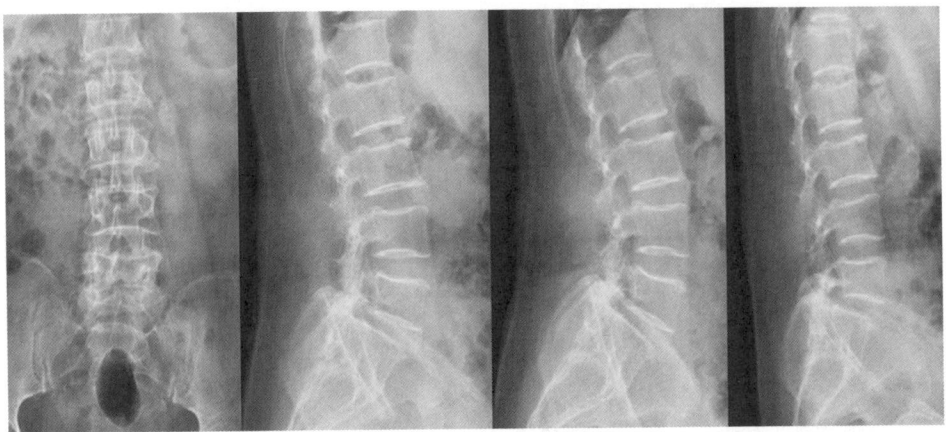

FIG. 6.39 Preoperative X-rays suggests L5 spondylolisthesis (I°) and mild degenerative scoliosis.

Case analysis

The symptoms of chronic lumbosacral pain were consistent with the symptoms of nerve root irritation in both lower limbs. So it was necessary to relieve nerve compression and rebuild segmental stability. For this patient, conventional MIS-TLIF and other minimally invasive surgery could be chosen. However, VBE assisted lumbar fusion was another option to minimize local soft tissue damage and bone structure destruction. Analyzing the dynamic position of X-ray, the reduction in segmental instability was not difficult. There was no sign of spontaneous fusion of the bilateral facet joints, so the unilateral VBE lumbar fusion could achieve satisfactory reduction.

Operative key points

This patient had a lumbosacral transitional vertebra, and the surgical segment could be considered as L5/S1. Since the working channel needed to be placed parallel to the intervertebral space to facilitate the implantation of the fusion cage, the iliac crest must be considered when performing VBE lumbar fusion. Therefore, for the case of the L5/S1 surgical segment, it was necessary to analyze the imaging examination comprehensively and carefully before the operation. In the case of the high iliac crest, the distance from lateral to the midline could be appropriately reduced, and the working channel could dock on the outside of the articular process to avoid the slide of trephine during the partial facetectomy. If necessary, the puncture guide needle could be pulled out, and the trephine could remove more articular process by moving the cannula inward. After the articular process was removed, the width of the exposed intervertebral disc could be observed to assess insertion of fusion cage. The cage mold could be introduced through the upper working channel of VBE cannula. If there was a bony structure obstructing the path, we could move the front end of the working sleeve to the outside. If the inner side of the mold was blocked by a bony structure, move the front end of the working sleeve to the outside to bypass the bony structure and reach the intervertebral disc. The U-shaped tip of the cannula should be monitored. If the cannula moved to outside too much, there is risk of nerve root injury. In such cases, it means that the operation space for lumbar fusion is not sufficient, and it was necessary to use tools such as a half trephine or laminectomy punch to remove more bony mass to obtain more operation space (Figure 6.40).

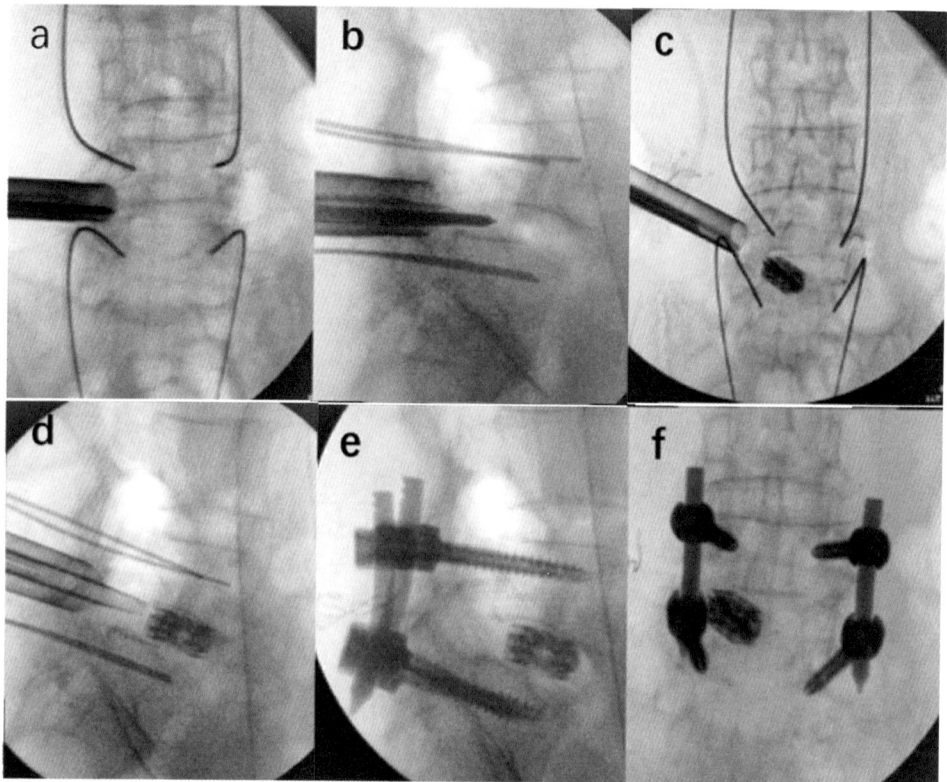

FIG. 6.40 X ray images during the surgery.
(a), (b) Placing the guidewire and working channel through the pedicle; (c), (d) decompress under the endoscope and cage placement; (e), (f) percutaneous pedicle screw placement.

Case 9
Abstract
The patient had pain in both lower limbs after a fall one year ago, and hip soreness (heavier on the right side) after walking for 300 m. These symptoms aggravated 1 month ago. After walking about 100 m, numbness of both lower limbs occurred and relieved after rest. The imaging examination revealed L4 spondylolisthesis (I°) and lumbar spinal stenosis. After evaluation, VBE endoscopic decompression, bone graft fusion, and internal fixation were performed under general anesthesia.

Patient information
Medical history: A 70-year-old female retiree complained of pain in both lower limbs

and intermittent claudication for one year, which was aggravated for more than one month. Previous medical history of severe osteoporosis.

Physical examination: Lumbar curvature existed. Lumbar spinous process tenderness and percussion tenderness (+). The straight leg raising test of the left lower limb was negative. Hypesthesia in the foot. Muscle strength of both lower limbs: iliopsoas muscle and extensor hallucis muscle were MRC grade 5; quadriceps, gastrocnemius, and tibialis anterior were MRC grade 3. Weakened knee jerk and Achilles's tendon reflexes. Pathological reflex (−).

Imaging examination: CT and MRI showed lumbar spinal stenosis and L4 spondylolisthesis (I°). MRN image showed no nerve root anomaly (Figures 6.41–6.43).

Preoperative diagnosis: Lumbar spondylolisthesis (I°, L4), lumbar spinal stenosis, osteoporosis.

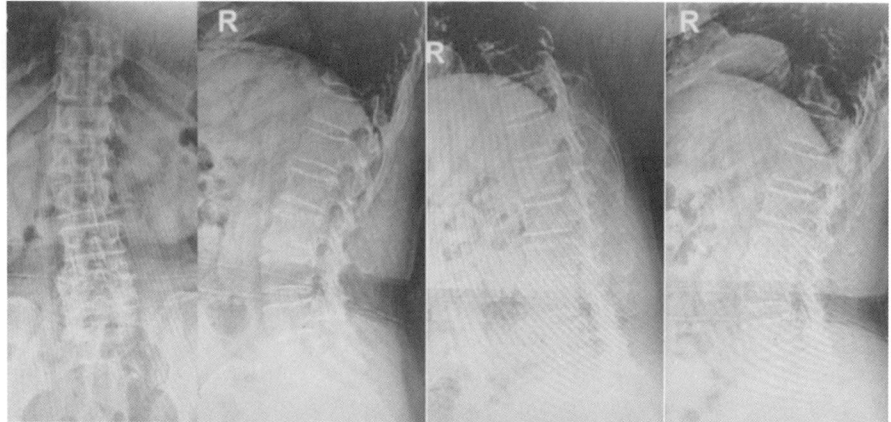

FIG. 6.41 Preoperative X-ray.

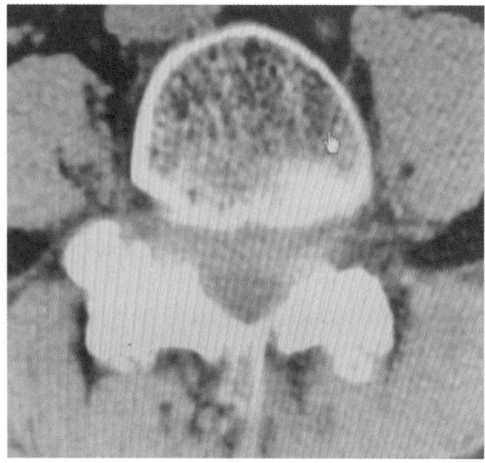

FIG. 6.42 Preoperative CT in transverse section.

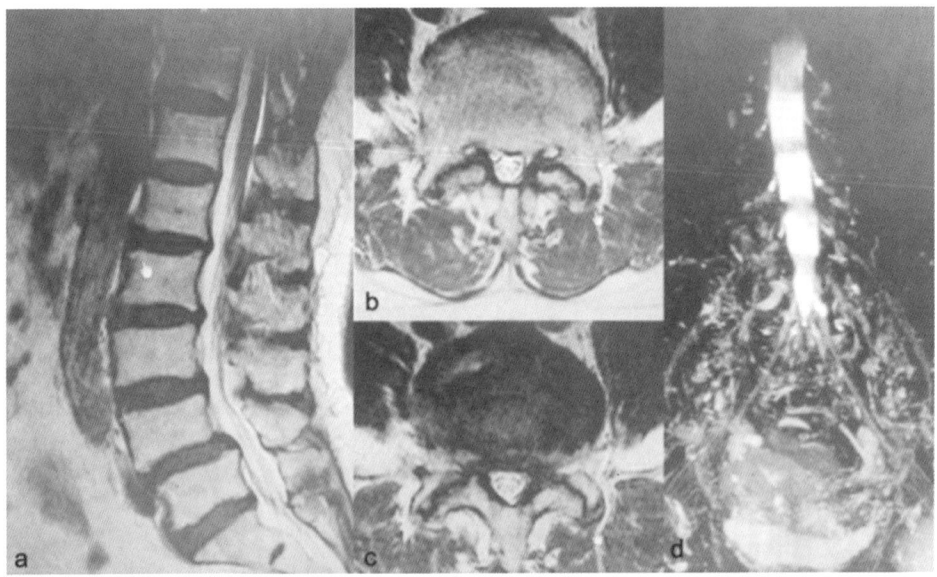

FIG. 6.43 Preoperative MRI and MRN.
(a) Sagittal section view; (b),(c) cross section view; (d) MRN image.

Case analysis

The main cause was L4 spondylolisthesis which resulted in stenosis of the corresponding level. The symptoms on the right side were more serious, so VBE lumbar fusion can be performed from the right side, and pedicle screws with cement augmentation can also be used for osteoporosis.

Operative key points

Preoperative CT showed that the patient had compensatory hyperosteogeny of the articular process due to L4 spondylolisthesis and segmental instability, which was obvious on the right side. For such patients with significant compensatory of the articular process, the puncture guide needle cannot puncture smoothly along the ventral side of the facet into the intervertebral disc. So it was difficult to guide and anchor the working cannula. At this time, the front end of the needle can be slightly biased to the caudal side and anchored in the upper posterior bone of the lower vertebral body. The trephine could be inserted after adjusting the working cannula by rotating clockwise/counterclockwise along the puncture guide needle. Attention should be paid to prevent pedicle damage caused by trephine. Due to the hyperosteogeny of the articular process, more bone should be removed by moving the working channel inward to obtain enough space for interbody fusion (Figures 6.44 and 6.45).

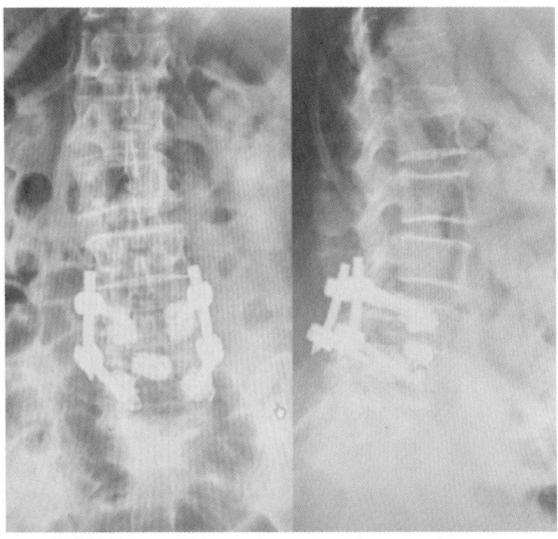

FIG. 6.44　X-ray at postoperative day 4.

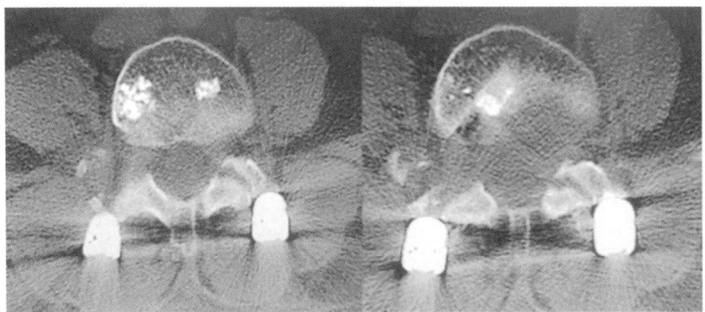

FIG. 6.45　CT in transverse section at postoperative day 3.

6.3　VBE Lumbar Fusion for Lumbar Instability

Case 10
Abstract

The patient complained of recurrent low back pain for more than two years, and the symptoms were significantly aggravated during weight bearing. Imaging examination revealed L4 instability and mild L4/5 disc herniation.

Patient information

Medical history: A 65-year-old male retiree complained of repeated low back pain for more than two years. There was previous history of hypertension, and blood pressure management was good with regular medication.

Physical examination: Lumbar physiological curvature degeneration. Normal sensation. The knee jerk and Achilles's tendon reflexes were normal. Pathological reflex (−).

Imaging examination: X-rays in the dynamic position suggested L4 instability (Figures 6.46). CT and MRI revealed L4/5 and L5/S1 disc herniation and mild spinal stenosis (Figures 6.47 and 6.48).

Preoperative diagnosis: Lumbar instability (L4), lumbar disc herniation (L4/5, L5/S1), hypertension.

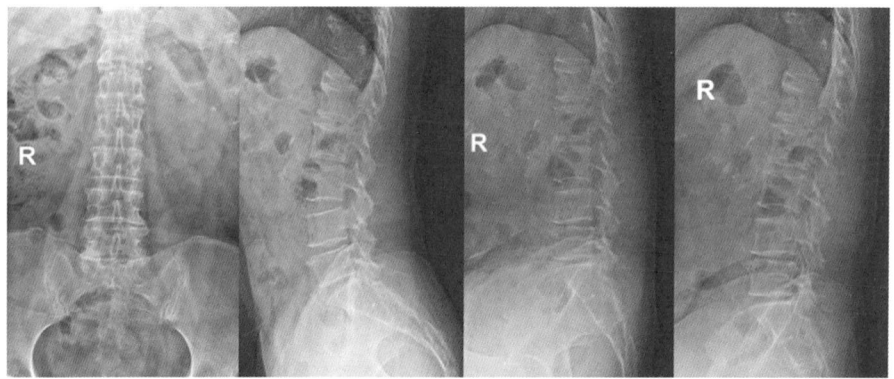

FIG. 6.46 X-ray shows L4 instability, narrowing of the intervertebral space at L4/5, L5/S1 segments.

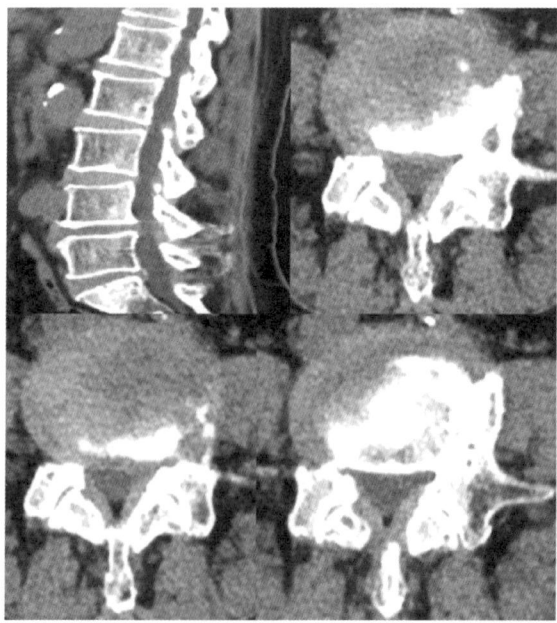

FIG. 6.47 CT shows L4/5 intervertebral disc herniation and lateral recess stenosis.

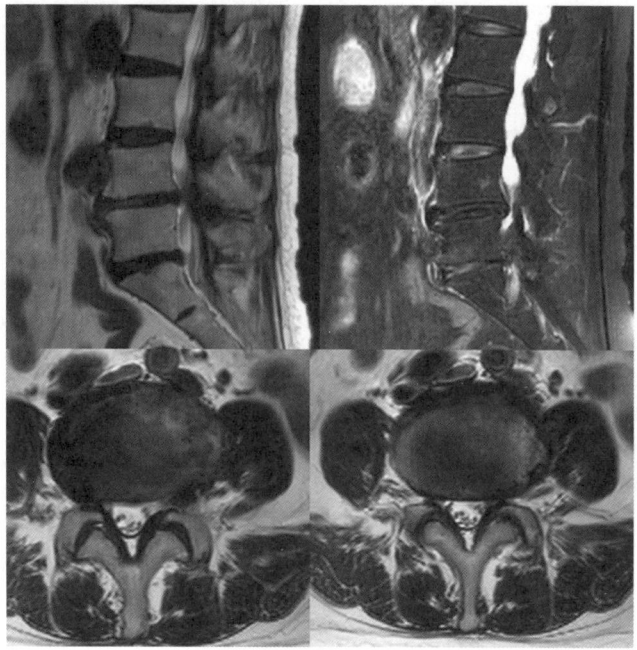

FIG. 6.48   MRI demonstrates L4/5 intervertebral disc herniation and lateral recess stenosis.

Case analysis

The patient complained of recurrent low back pain, which worsened during weight bearing and was partly relieved after rest. Combined with X-rays in the dynamic position, CT, and MRI, the symptoms were consistent with lumbar instability. Lumbar fusion and internal fixation were suitable for such patients. Because decompression was not required, VBE lumbar fusion could directly complete the bone graft fusion and internal fixation without exposing the spinal canal, which is very suitable for such case. Therefore, to some extent, the VBE technique shows some advantages which are similar to oblique lumbar interbody fusion (OLIF).

Operative key points

When removing the articular process, there is no need to remove too many bony fragments on the inner side. Bone graft fusion can be performed without exposing the spinal canal to avoid the irritation of hemorrhage to the dural sac and the occurrence of dural sac adhesion, which is also one of the advantages of the V-shape bichannel endoscopy (Figures 6.49 and 6.50).

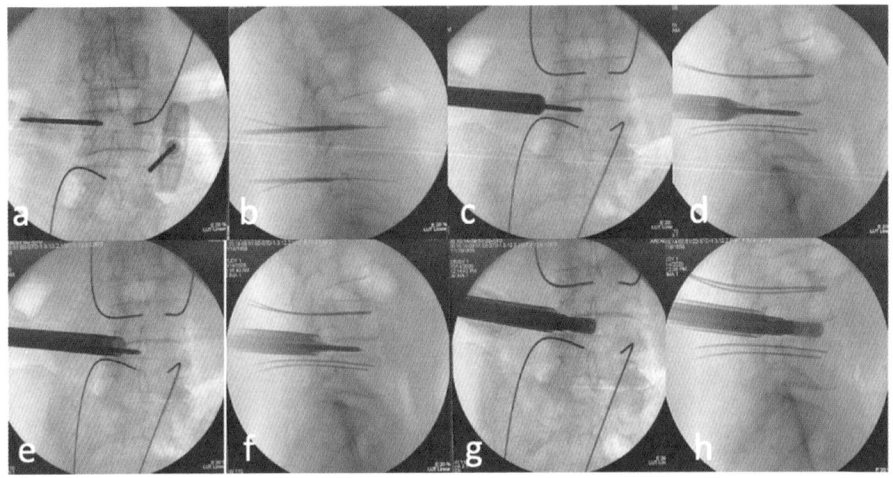

FIG. 6.49 Pictures of intraoperative operation.
(a),(b) Placing the guidewire through the pedicle; (c),(d) the sequential dilators were passed through the soft tissue and a working channel was inserted; (e),(f) partial facetectomy using VBE system; (g),(h) decompress and interbody fusion.

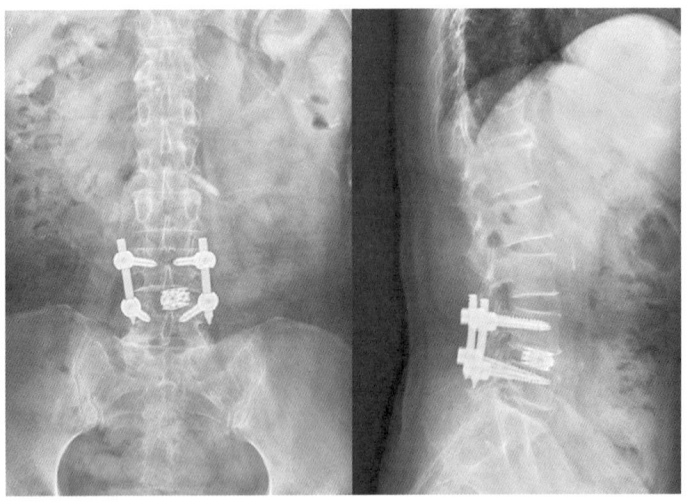

FIG. 6.50 X-ray at postoperative day 3 shows the internal fixation was in a good position.

6.4 VBE Lumbar Fusion for Recurrent Lumbar Disc Herniation

Case 11
Abstract
The patient underwent percutaneous transforaminal endoscopic lumbar discectomy

in our institution about 20 months ago due to lumbar disc herniation, and the symptoms relieved after the operation. However, about a month ago, radiating pain recurred on the right lower extremity. The MRI showed that the original operation segment had recurred intervertebral disc herniation. Considering factors such as age and patient's demands, VBE endoscopic decompression, bone graft fusion, and internal fixation were performed under general anesthesia.

Patient information

Medical history: A 67-year-old male retiree complained of low back pain and right lower limb pain for one month. It was about 20 months after percutaneous transforaminal endoscopic lumbar discectomy. No particular previous medical history.

Physical examination: Antalgic gait. No deformity. Lumbar physiological curvature degeneration. Limitation of lumbar motion with provocative pain. Lumbar spinous process tenderness and percussion tenderness (+). The straight leg raising test of the right lower limb was positive at 60°, and the augment test was positive. Hypesthesia in the posterior outer side of the right crus and the right instep. Muscle strength of both lower limbs: iliopsoas muscle and extensor hallucis muscle were MRC grade 5 (left) and grade 4 (right); tibialis anterior and quadriceps were MRC grade 5.Weakened knee jerk and Achilles's tendon reflexes. Pathological reflex (−).

Imaging examination: CT and MRI showed L4/5 intervertebral disc herniation on the right side and the corresponding segment of the nerve compression. MRN image showed no nerve root anomaly (Figures 6.51–6.53).

Preoperative diagnosis: Lumbar disc herniation (L4/5), post lumbar spine surgery status.

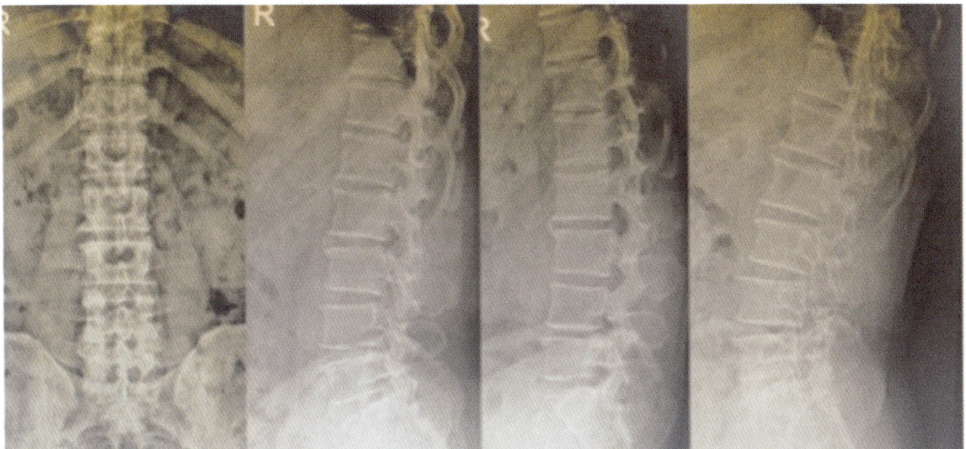

FIG. 6.51 Preoperative X-ray shows lumbar physiological curvature degeneration, narrowing of the intervertebral space at L4/5.

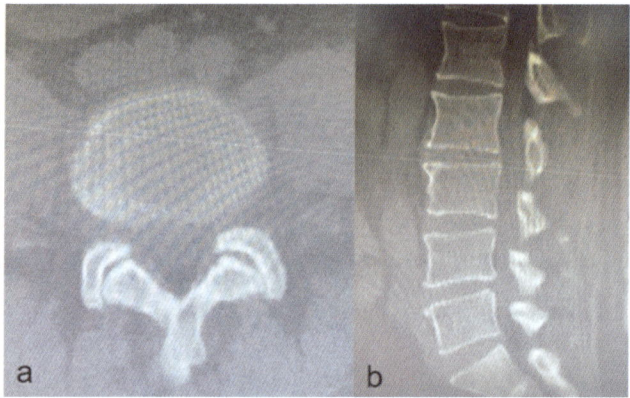

FIG. 6.52 CT shows massive lumbar disc herniation.
(a) Cross section view; (b) sagittal section view.

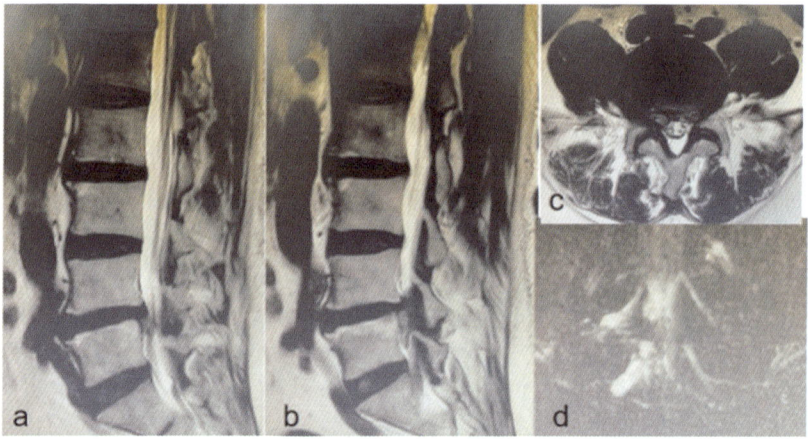

FIG. 6.53 MRI demonstrates L4/5 disc herniation and downward prolapse.
(a),(b) Sagittal section view; (c) cross section view; (d) MRN image.

Case analysis

The patient was diagnosed with postoperative recurrence of lumbar disc herniation. According to the preoperative imaging examination, there is a certain degree of lumbar instability. Combined with the patient's age and long-term effect, VBE lumbar fusion was selected.

Operative key points

When performing facet joint resection for a narrow intervertebral space, attention should be paid to avoid nerve root damage. On the one hand, the puncture guide needle could anchor in the upper part of the inferior vertebral body' posterior bone structures. In addition, the working cannula should be placed as close as possible to the caudal end and parallel to the intervertebral space. Since the patient has undergone surgery on the same segment, scars and soft tissue adhesions were inevitable. Therefore, it was necessary to carefully identify soft tissues and nerves during the operation. Rough operations of instruments should be avoided. At the same time, decompress procedure should be carried out from the ventral side to the dorsal side, or from the inner disc to the dorsal side. It would be safer and reduced the probability of nerve injury (Figures 6.54–6.57).

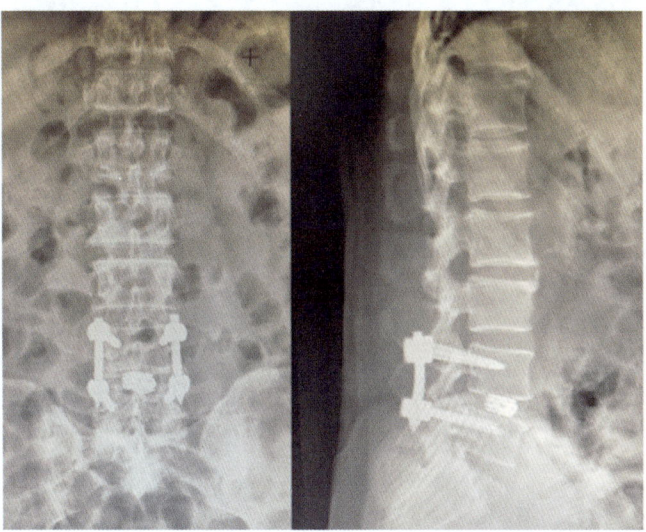

FIG. 6.54 X-ray after the operation shows the internal fixation, and the fusion cage was in a good position.

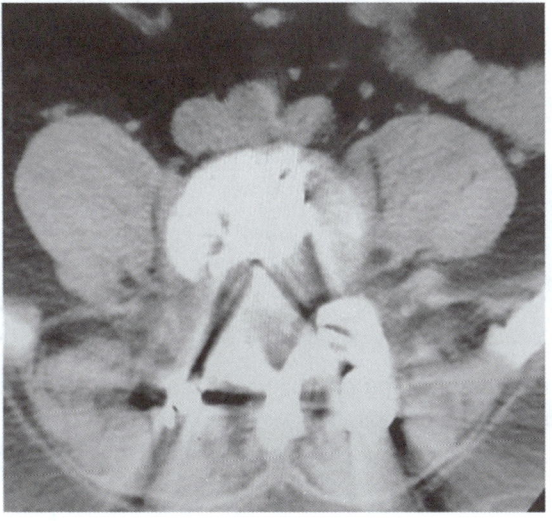

FIG. 6.55 CT images (5 days after the operation) in transverse section showing the internal fixation's position was satisfactory.

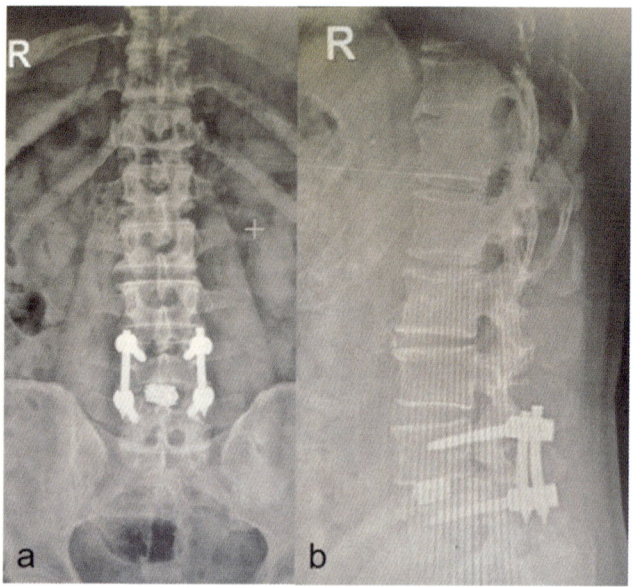

FIG. 6.56 X-ray image at 3 months after surgery.
(a) Anteroposterior view; (b) lateral view.

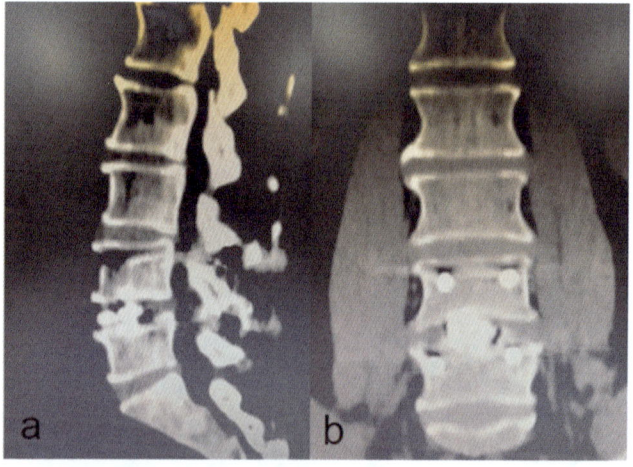

FIG. 6.57 Three months after the operation, CT shows that the fusion cage was in a good position without sinking or migration.
(a) Sagittal section view; (b) coronal section view.

Case 12
Abstract
The patient accepted percutaneous transforaminal endoscopic lumbar discectomy

4 months ago due to L4/5 disc herniation. Two months after surgery, low back pain recurred with numbness and pain in the left lower extremity. The MRI showed L4/5 intervertebral disc herniation on the right side. The patient had severe obesity (weight 110 kg, BMI 33.9), which was a risk factor for recurrence. Therefore, he requested fusion and internal fixation surgery, and VBE endoscopic decompression, bone graft fusion, and internal fixation were performed under general anesthesia.

Patient information

Medical history: A 30-year-old male employee complained of recurrence of lumbar disc herniation and numbness and pain in the left lower extremity for 2 months.

Physical examination: No deformity. Lumbar physiological curvature degeneration. The surgical incision in the lumbosacral area healed well. Lumbar spinous process tenderness and percussion tenderness (−). Hypesthesia in the outer side of the left leg. The straight leg raising test of the left leg was positive at 50°, and the augment test was positive. The straight leg raising test of the right lower limb was negative. Muscle strength of both lower limbs: iliopsoas muscle, quadriceps, gastrocnemius, and extensor hallucis muscle were MRC grade 5; tibialis anterior were MRC grade 3 (left) and grade 5 (right). The knee jerk and Achilles's tendon reflection were normal. Pathological reflex (−).

Imaging examination: X-ray showed mild scoliosis and degeneration of the lumbar spine. MRI showed huge protrusion of lumbar intervertebral disc (L4/5, left side) and lumbar spinal stenosis (L4/5) (Figures 6.58 and 6.59).

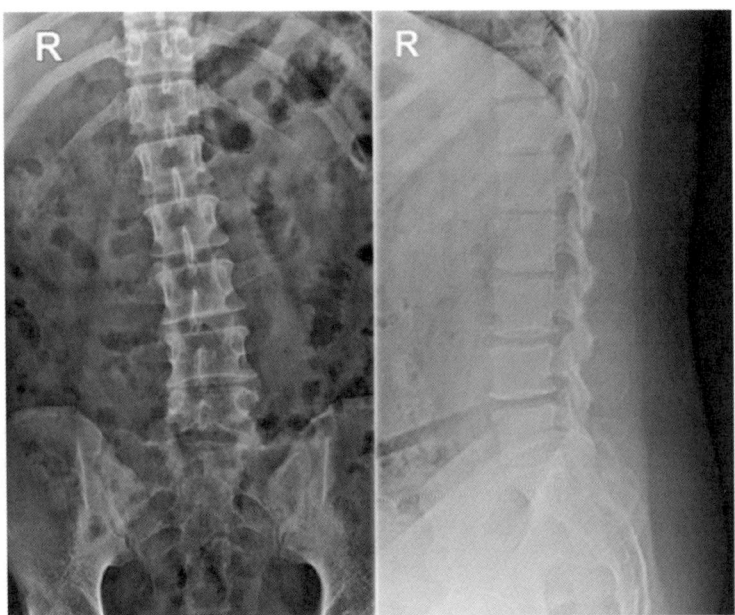

FIG. 6.58 Preoperative X-ray shows the lumbar curvature was straight and compensatory scoliosis.

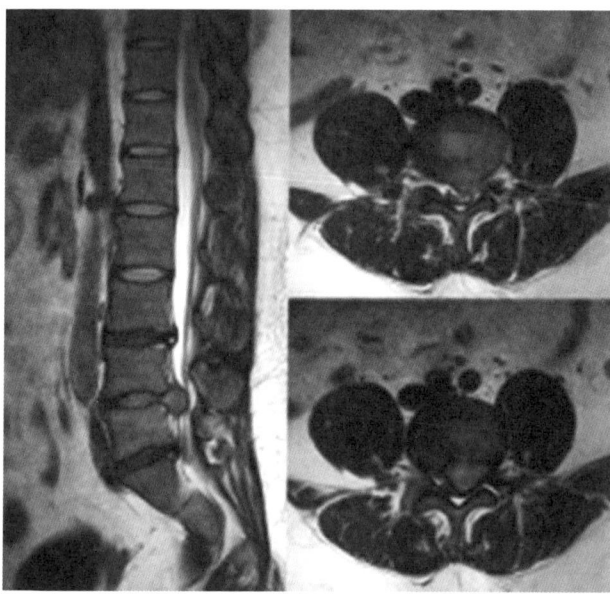

FIG. 6.59 MRI shows huge protrusion of lumbar intervertebral disc (L4/5, left side) with spinal stenosis.

Preoperative diagnosis: Lumbar disc herniation (L4/5, left side), lumbar spinal stenosis (L4/5), post lumbar surgery status, severe obesity.

Case analysis

The patient was severely obese with a higher risk of recurrence after discectomy without fusion. The patient fully understood the situation and requested interbody fusion. Traditional open surgery for this patient would be very traumatic. MIS-TLIF was challenging because of the limited length of working channel, while, the VBE system was suitable for such a case. The length of the VBE working cannula was enough for the surgery and provided the surgeon with a clear view of the surgical field. The VBE assisted interbody fusion would ensure the surgical safety and reduce trauma.

Operative key points

To avoid nerve damage, the surgeon can first perform the intervertebral fusion procedure and then replace the VBE system with a traditional single-port endoscopic system for decompression (Figures 6.60 and 6.61).

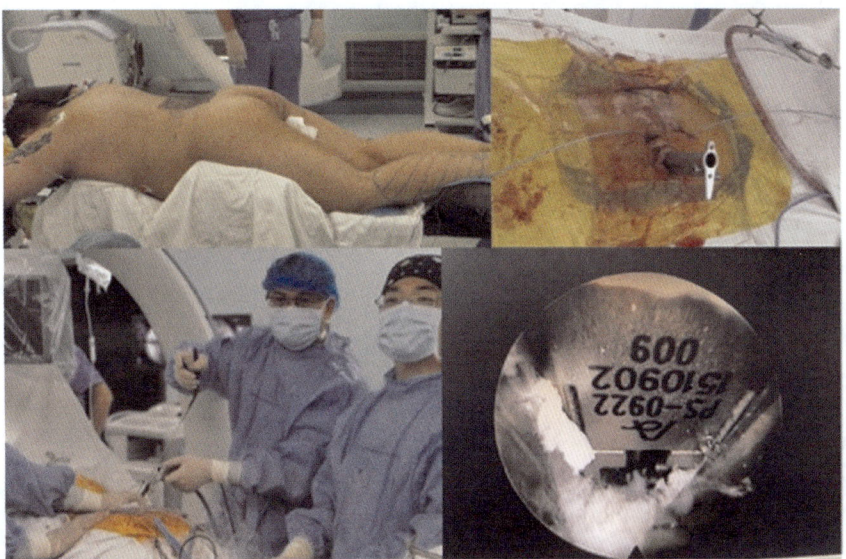

FIG. 6.60 VBE lumbar fusion for severely obese patients. The limited working channel length will increase the difficulty of MIS-TLIF, while the length of the VBE working cannula was enough for this surgery.

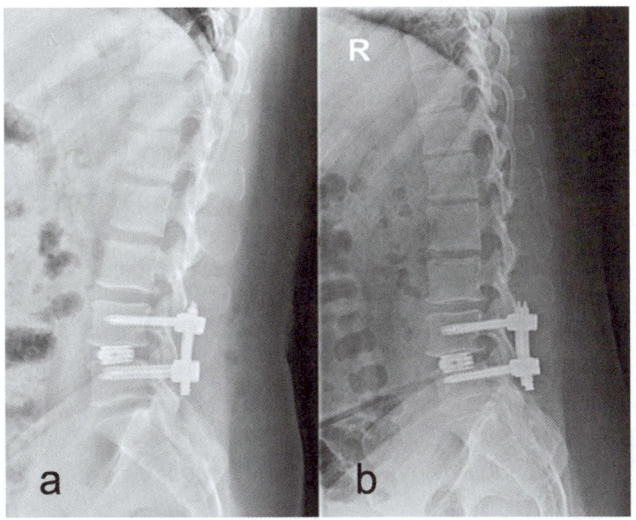

FIG. 6.61 Postoperative X-ray examinations.
(a) One month after operation, the lateral X-ray shows that the internal fixation position was satisfactory; (b) one year after operation, the lateral X-ray shows that the position of internal fixation and cage was good.

Chapter 7

Lumbar Surgery Rehabilitation

Section Editors

Amanda Ferland, MD
Xin Zhang, MD
Chun Feng, MD
Huang Yan, MD
Xun Yang, MD

7.1 Introduction

The surgeon's decision to perform surgery on the lumbar spine is multi-faceted, as is explained in detail in this book. As rehabilitation specialists, we are spending large amounts of time with our patients, getting to know their histories, their goals, and their lives. Low back pain occurs in a very large percentage of the human population, and there are significant amounts of research that show that the majority of us will experience low back pain (LBP) at least once in our lives [1, 2].

However, as you likely know by now, most of us do not need surgery. Those that do require surgery of any kind are likely doing so because there was either a significant acute injury, or there has been a chronic debilitating injury that has only gotten worse. In the case of the latter situation, most countries/cultures will attempt conservative treatment multiple times (or for multiple months/years) for chronic LBP before they will consider surgery. So, for those patients who have been dealing with chronic pain, a surgery like those mentioned in this book needs to be considered the very best and last option, and will therefore likely require more awareness and a unique approach from the rehabilitation specialist.

Microdiscectomy is usually performed on a younger, more active population, due to the fact that "young discs" have higher hydration levels, which can lead to higher intradiscal pressure, causing herniation of nuclear material into the epidural space. As has been stated in other parts of this book, minimally invasive microdiscectomy causes little damage to the surrounding tissue, and should therefore allow for more aggressive rehabilitation [3]. Other surgeries on the low back, such as lumbar fusion can cause more damage to the surrounding tissue, but the surgical techniques discussed here are designed to help minimize soft tissue damage.

This chapter was designed to provide you with the best evidence for all patients with low back pain (LBP) and provide you with specific evidence-based practice for those who have had or will have these types of surgery. We will begin by introducing the guidelines from the Academy of Orthopaedic Physical Therapy (AOPT) related to LBP. These guidelines were first published in 2012, and have proven to be the foremost authority on diagnosing and understanding LBP in a rehabilitation setting. These guidelines also have a revision to be published in 2021.

Once we have introduced the guidelines, it is important to understand the rehabilitation patterns that most closely relate to patients who will likely have lumbar surgery. Patients with patterns that are labeled LBP with referred pain and LBP with radiating pain could have surgery, so it is important to understand the presentation and treatment for patients with these patterns.

The next section will provide information about preoperative rehabilitation and patient education. Research has found that, in certain circumstances, a small amount of treatment before surgery can provide better outcomes after surgery. We will then discuss postoperative complications, which are few but can influence our rehabilitation outcomes. Therefore, we need to be aware of these possibilities.

We will then spend the rest of this chapter providing specific rehabilitation timelines, goals, education, and treatment for each phase of postoperative care for different types of surgery.

7.2 Low Back Pain Clinical Practice Guideline

The Orthopedic Section of the American Physical Therapy Society has been collecting experts to compile clinical practice guidelines since before the first published guideline in 2008. Since that time, guidelines (and revisions of guidelines) have been published for nearly every joint of the body, as well as some post-operative pathologies.

The Low Back Pain clinical practice guideline was originally published in 2012, with the revision draft completed and likely approved for publication in 2021 [4, 5].

The original guideline provided moderate evidence supporting classifying low back pain into 5 distinctive patterns:

(1) Low Back Pain with Mobility Deficits
(2) Low Back Pain with Movement Coordination Impairments
(3) Low Back Pain with Referred Lower Extremity Pain
(4) Low Back Pain with Radiating Pain
(5) Low Back Pain with Related Generalized Pain

See Table 7.1 for summary statements related to these patterns.

Of these 5 recognized patterns, it is likely that patients requiring lumbar surgery present with either the Low Back Pain with Referred Lower Extremity Pain, Low Back Pain with Radiating Pain, or some combination of these two patterns. Being able to understand the differences between these presentations/patterns makes it easier for rehabilitation specialists to evaluate, choose the best treatment, and monitor the outcomes of these patients.

TAB. 7.1 Low back pain: Clinical practice guidelines 2012.

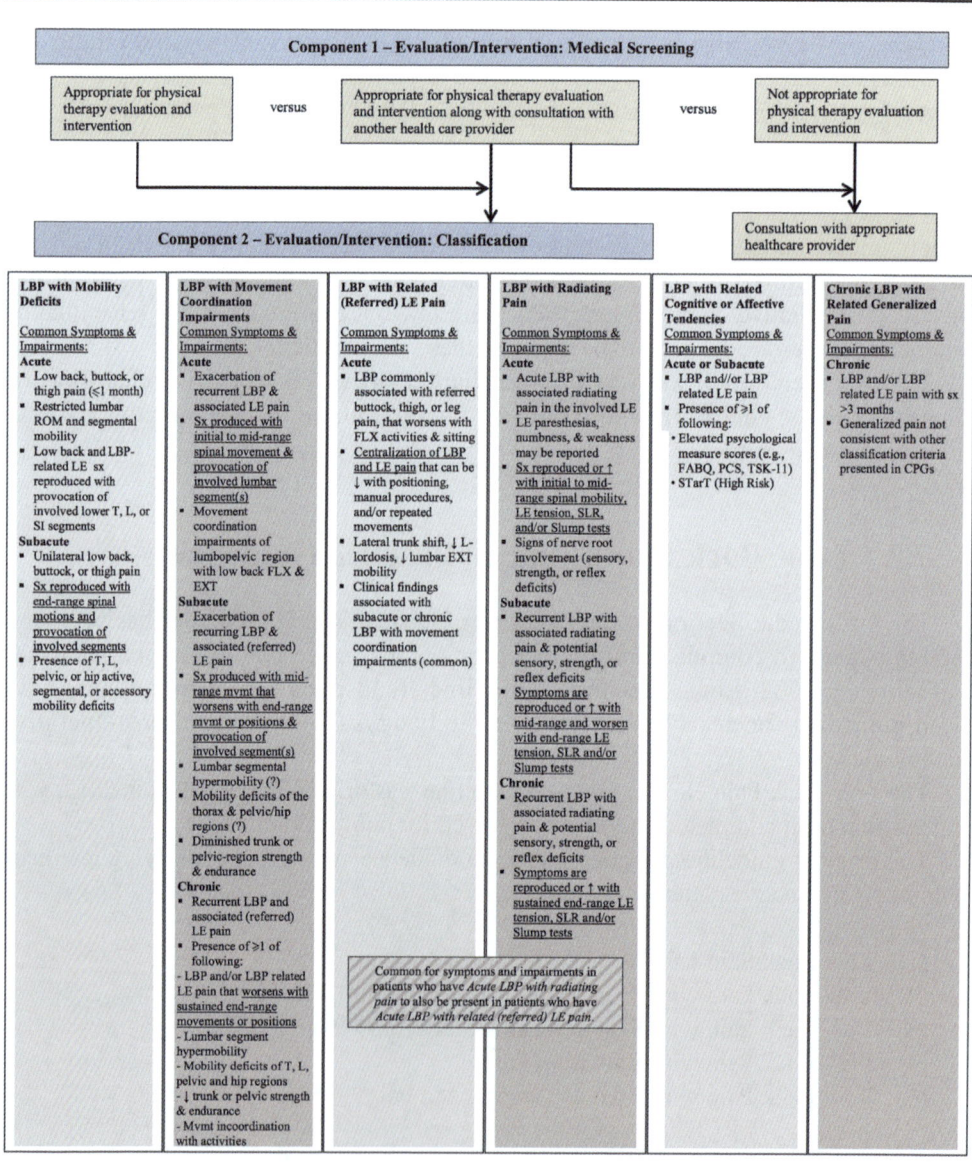

Low back pain with referred lower extremity pain can often be classified as an injury to the intervertebral disc. Most cases of disc injury can be treated with conservative treatment, which often focuses on exercises, manual therapy, and/or traction to promote centralization of lower extremity symptoms.

Low back pain with radiating pain is often classified as an injury to one or more nerve roots in the lumbar spine. This leads to a sharp pain "like a line" down the leg, as well as possible paresthesia, numbness, and/or weakness in the leg. Nerve root involvement can be treated by conservative care as well, with treatment including nerve mobilization, soft tissue mobilization (STM) around nerve pathways, and possibly traction.

Once these pattern presentations have been treated, and the patient reports decreased lower extremity referred or radiating pain, the patient will often still need treatment that falls into the low back pain with movement coordination impairments pattern.

Low back pain with movement coordination impairments pattern usually presents as a primary pattern for patients with chronic low back pain that do not have radiating or referred lower extremity pain and report pain with back movements. This group can demonstrate increased mobility of specific lumbar spine segments and pain during mid-range motions or prolonged positions of the low back. Treatment for this pattern focuses on therapeutic exercises to improve trunk strength and endurance, as well as neuromuscular reeducation of functional activities.

Many patients following lumbar surgery will report significant relief of any previous referred or radiating pain but will continue to present with decreased coordination of the trunk and lower body. Therefore, treatment focus will eventually look very similar to what is recommended for our patients following the low back pain with movement coordination impairment pattern.

Much of the treatment section of this chapter will go into detail regarding this treatment approach.

7.3 Preoperative Rehabilitation

Please note: Many hospitals/insurances do not provide preoperative rehabilitation care. If the patient cannot receive this instruction/ information before surgery, it can be provided immediately after surgery as well.

Patient Education

Preoperative rehabilitation for most surgeries focuses on patient education. Patient education for lumbar surgery includes helping the patient understand the surgical process and timing of hospitalization. Some surgeons will ask the patient not to perform any bending, lifting, or twisting for 6 weeks or more, depending on the procedure. Most surgeons will restrict heavy lifting (>10 kg) for 12 weeks or more. These movement restrictions need to be understood by the patient before surgery. Instructing patients on proper wound care techniques, and the importance of keeping the wound clean and dry after surgery are also helpful preoperatively.

Functional Movement Instruction

Once the therapist understands if the surgeon is providing movement restrictions, they can instruct the patient on proper movement techniques. Depending on patient's symptoms and irritability level preoperatively, the therapist can instruct the patient on bed mobility to prevent twisting and sleeping positions that will put less stress on the wound. They can also review performing sit-to-stand with a flat back (no bending in lumbar spine) and walking with an upright posture (Figure 7.1). If appropriate, the therapist can consider reviewing proper lifting technique, though it is unlikely the patient will be doing any lifting for several months after the surgery.

Performing regular cardiovascular exercises preoperatively has also been found to improve outcomes and decrease hospital length of stay [6].

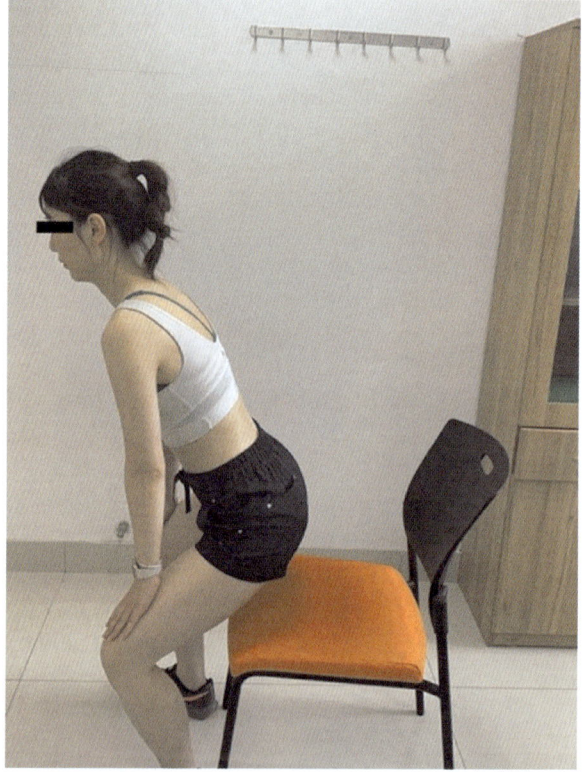

FIG. 7.1 Sit to stand with neutral spine and flat back.

Core Recruitment Instruction

Multiple studies [3, 7] have reported that patients who injure their lumbar spine demonstrate decreased recruitment of the lumbar multifidus muscle, especially at the level of pain and/or injury.

A randomized controlled study by Rowley and colleagues [7] in 2019 assessed multifidus and transverse abdominus (deeper trunk muscles) recruitment, compared to erector spinae and more superficial abdominal muscle recruitment, in patients with low back pain. Conclusions were similar to previous studies and found that deeper trunk muscles were not recruited well in patients with chronic low back pain, and the multifidus had actually atrophied at the level of pain/injury. The authors also concluded that when these deeper muscles did not contract with arm and leg movements, the superficial muscles were less likely to contract to stabilize the back.

Sions J.M. et al. [8] looked at cross-sectional measurements of the multifidi, erector spinae, psoas, and quadratus lumborum in 53 older adults with chronic low back pain and matched 49 adults without pain. They found that those with chronic low back pain, especially women, demonstrated up to 54% fat in their multifidi, with a smaller amount in their erector spinae. The psoas and quadratus lumborum were unchanged and similar to their matched controls.

Studies like these have been reviewed, and rehabilitation specialists have come to some very important conclusions. Paul Hodges and others [9] have theorized that the change in fiber type is likely mediated by neural changes from immune response, i.e. inflammation. Exercise has been found to target immune system activity in tissues in a positive way, influencing peripheral input from the spine and pathological central nervous system plasticity. This can be an encouraging information and research to share with our patients regarding the importance of exercise after surgery.

Paul Hodges and Lieven Danneels provided a clinical commentary in 2019 that assessed the lower trunk muscles of patients with low back pain at "different time points, observations, and mechanisms" [10]. They summarized that there are two sections of multifidus muscles. Deep multifidus cross about 2 segments, whereas more superficial erector spinae and multifidus cross up to 5 segments. Deep multifidus provide compression with limited extension movement, while superficial muscles produce spine extension. When injury to the lumbar spine occurs, superficial muscles will increase activation (which can lead to decreased flexion tolerance), and deep multifidus muscle activation cannot occur. This can then lead to atrophy of the multifidi, as well as the possibility of the multifidus being used only as a back extensor.

However, it has been found that gentle activation of the deep multifidus can restore their recruitment and improve muscle cross-sectional area in the acute phase. This is especially true if early intervention can be provided.

As one progresses into the subacute phase, strength training helps to increase the size and number of deep muscle fibers, decreasing the use of superficial fibers.

As patients move into the chronic phase of low back pain, fatty and fibrotic changes become more consistent. If this has occurred with our patients who have a microdiscectomy, we need to help the patient first establish activation of the deep multifidus, and then provide resistance training to restructure the musculature. We show examples of multifidus assessment and treatment in Figure 7.2.

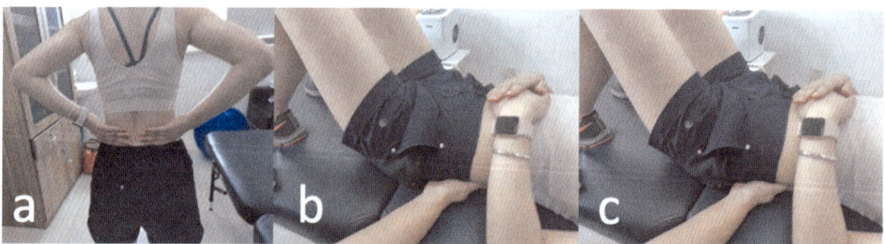

FIG. 7.2 Multifidus assessment and treatment.

(a) Multifidus palpation: place fingers on either side of the low back, just lateral to the spinous process, and bend forward just slightly. Multifidus should turn on at each level of the spine; (b) Multifidus palpation with neutral spine: therapist and/or patient palpates multifidus in supine position on one side of spine; (c) Neutral spine instruction: therapist instructs patient to gently press back down into hand. This movement should come from pelvis, a small posterior pelvic tilt. Multifidus and transverse abdominal muscle contraction should be felt with therapist/patient's hand.

As stated in Hodges' commentary, "Rehabilitation of LBP is likely to require a multifaceted approach that includes consideration of multiple interacting 'bottom-up' and 'top-down' biological mechanisms that interact with the neural processing of nociception and pain and sensorimotor control of the spine." In rehabilitation terms, with this patient population, we need to help reeducate the deep muscles around the spine with larger functional movements to help rebuild a normal nervous system response, as well as normal muscular tissue [11].

Another research study out of Taiwan [12] looked at patients who had minimally invasive surgery (including lumbar fusion) focused on trunk control (forwardreaching and center-of-pressure) and compared them to controls one month after surgery. They found that this patient population continued to show decreased trunk control one month after surgery, despite significant pain relief and improved function.

Following fusion, it is also important to keep in mind that neutral spine education helps to minimize strain on surgical areas, as well as surrounding areas. Levels above and below with fused vertebrae will attempt to compensate, and this can lead to complications, like sacroiliac pain, described later in this chapter. Providing neutral spine education can help the fused area work better with the surrounding areas [13].

Educating the patient about these muscle groups early in the rehabilitation process, as well as providing instruction on how to reinstate contraction is a large focus of rehabilitation treatment.

Neuroscience Education

Preoperative neuroscience education can also be very helpful, especially for patients who might be suffering from anxiety or fear from acute symptoms or the chronic low back pain experience. It is important for the patient to understand that the decision to have the surgery was the right decision, and we want to confirm that they are not questioning this decision.

While it is outside the scope of this chapter, nervous system physiology and pathways can also be part of this discussion. Helping the patient better understand peripheral nerve sensitization and the effects of surgical experiences and environmental issues on nerve sensitivity can often be comforting and important knowledge. AdriaanLouw and colleagues studied the effect of neuroscience education preoperatively in a group of patients with chronic low back pain, and found more significant positive effects on pain, catastrophization, and physical movement outcomes following surgery when compared to those patients who did not receive this education [14].

7.4 Patient Education

We understand that each patient is unique and will likely have different experiences and restrictions regarding function. Therefore, certain statements might be helpful to provide during the process.

(1) During therapy, a physical therapist will teach you exercises to use muscles in that area to help support your back with normal movements that you do throughout your day.

They will also discuss your goals regarding what types of activities that you would like to return to. For example, do you like to swim? Your therapist will progress exercises that allow you to return to swimming. The same can be said for other sports or work activities.

(2) Recovery from each surgery is different. Some patients return to full activity in 4–6 weeks while other patients require more time. Your physical therapist can help you safely begin the process of returning to normal activities.

(3) A systematic review of over 430 000 patients found that movement, with the help of a physical therapist, following minimally invasive spinal surgery provided no risk to the patient, and actually decreased the possibility of complications [15].

Therefore, if you want to get back to the activities that you did before surgery with minimal pain and greater movement, it is important to include physical therapy in your recovery.

7.5 Surgical Complications

Microdiscectomy

Complications from microdiscectomy are generally rare and will be discussed in more detail in other parts of this book. However, it is important for rehabilitation specialists to have basic knowledge of complications that they should be watching for during our treatment process. Therefore, we will briefly discuss several things to be watching for during rehabilitation.

It is important to note that most research before 2015 reports no difference in complications between "open" and percutaneous microdiscectomy [16]. However, a more recent meta-analysis from 2020 does report that percutaneous endoscopic lumbar discectomy (PELD) has decreased overall risk of complications, reporting 5.8% overall complications for PELD, compared to 16% for open microdiscectomy [17].

The most common complication is infection, with infection rates anywhere from 0.7% to 12%. Postoperative hematoma can also occur, but rates are only about 1% [16]. Treatment for infection or hematoma is usually outside of our job responsibilities, but assessing wound healing and instructing the patient to follow up with their surgeon or another doctor who can assist is very appropriate.

Injury to nerve root and/or new or worsening neurological deficit at level of surgery is serious but rare complications, with reported rates of 0.5%–3% [18]. It is likely that the surgeon will be aware of this complication before referral to you for treatment. Many patients will present with some residual neurological symptoms, and this should be evaluated during our post-operative evaluation. Myotomal and dermatomal symptoms previous to surgery could still be present to a smaller extent following surgery, especially as soft tissue around the disc and/or nerve root continue to heal. Helping to improve nerve and soft tissue mobility is an important part of postoperative treatment. As treatment continues, it is very important that you assess and reassess neurological symptoms. If the patient is reporting increased nerve pain, lower extremity weakness, or sensation changes, these things need to be reported to their surgeon as soon as possible.

Lumbar Fusion

A meta-analysis out of China [19] found that minimally invasive lumbar fusion "was highly associated with shorter length of hospital stay, less blood loss, and fewer complications."

As with microdiscectomy, wound infection appears to be the most common complication (9%) [18]. Therefore, assessing the wound during initial treatment is recommended, as it was following other lumbar surgeries.

Another meta-analysis [20] with 6699 patients undergoing minimally invasive lumbar fusion found that postoperative radiculitis was the primary complication. This is a complication that we must consider with our patients. The evaluation must include nerve tension assessment, as well as myotome and dermatome assessment. It is likely that these symptoms will decrease in 6–12 weeks, and patient education regarding this timeline is important. Many patients will experience some radicular symptoms that can feel similar to what they experienced before surgery, and this can be very scary for patients. From this author's familiarity with this situation, helping the patient understand this possibility, but providing cognitive behavioral therapy and encouragement to increase functional mobility has proven to provide positive outcomes. As stated with microdiscectomy, if the patient is experiencing an overall increase in lower extremity weakness or decreased sensation, this needs to be reported to surgeon as soon as possible.

From this author's experience, sacroiliac joint (SIJ) dysfunction can be the most difficult and debilitating complication following spinal fusion. We will discuss this more in detail later in this chapter, but it is important to consider how the patient's mechanics will change following lumbar fusion, which can cause increased strain on the pelvis, and this often leads to pain.

7.6 Postoperative Evaluation

Initial postoperative evaluation could occur in an inpatient setting on the same day as surgery or as an outpatient on the same day or several days (or even weeks) after surgery.

As discussed previously, the patient's function previous to surgery is a very important predictor of outcomes, as well as the aggressiveness of treatment. This includes understanding patient history and their activity level before surgery. Patients who have experienced chronic low back pain will require a different approach due to likelihood of deconditioning and possible generalized pain pattern presentation (as discussed earlier in this chapter).

Post-operative evaluation should consider a basic neurological evaluation, assessing for continued possible involvement of dermatomes and myotomes, leading to weakness and sensation changes. These changes could lead to difficulty with basic movement patterns.

One should always consider functional mobility assessment first. This will initially include bed mobility, supine-to-sit, and transfers. The amount of assistance the patient requires needs to be documented for function, and more importantly, safety.

If the patient can tolerate these basic movements, the rehabilitation specialist can then assess sit-to-stand, standing, and walking tolerance. More advanced movement patterns such as bending, lifting, and twisting will be assessed at a later time.

Functional assessment can help the clinician focus on appropriate further objective measurements. For instance, if they demonstrate decreased sit-to-stand tolerance, assessment should include knee and hip extension manual muscle testing. If they report lower extremity nerve symptoms with dorsiflexion during walking, one should assess sciatic nerve mobility. One should also consider the possibility of dural tension. If the patient has a history of chronic low back pain, assessing multifidus and transverse abdominal muscle endurance using something like Shirley Sahrmann trunk graded assessment (Figure 7.3) is absolutely necessary [21].

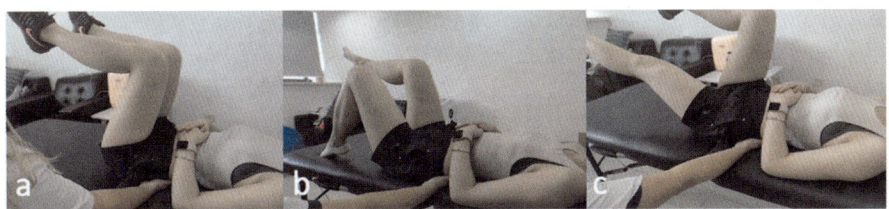

FIG. 7.3 Shirley Sahrmann trunk graded assessment.
(a) Shirley Sahrmann graded trunk assessment starting position; (b) Example of progression of trunk assessment; (c) Example of progression of trunk assessment.

7.7 Postoperative Rehabilitation Principles

Microdiscectomy

Research regarding timing to begin rehabilitation following microdiscectomy has been somewhat inconsistent. Most research suggests that intensive therapy before 4 weeks post-operatively did not provide any added benefit when compared to rehabilitation starting at 4–6 weeks. A systematic review of 22 low-quality studies (2503 patients) comparing different types of rehabilitation (multidisciplinary, strengthening, stretching, graded activity) found that it did not matter what type of treatment was provided, as long as something was provided starting 4–6 weeks after surgery. Functional outcomes and pain were significantly better in those who received rehabilitation versus those who did not, or those given education only [22]. The most recent clinical practice guideline did find one lower quality RCT by Ozkara *et al.* examining 30 patients following microdiscectomy and compared a general exercise program beginning immediately after surgery to a control group. The general exercise group had greater improvement in disability at 6 and 12 weeks, and greater improvement in pain at 12 weeks.

Lumbar Fusion

Most research looking at timing to begin treatment after lumbar fusion recommends rehabilitation starts immediately following surgery, especially to help establish a walking program and provide cognitive behavioral therapy as soon as possible [6]. However, similar to recommendations after microdiscectomy, consistent (2–3 times a week) treatment does not need to begin until 3 months postoperatively. Oestergaard L. *et al.* [23], did an excellent study in Spine that found that starting consistent rehabilitation at 6 weeks versus 12 weeks did not provide an added benefit. Some protocols even state that 8 visits are all that is required between 3 and 6 months postoperatively [6, 24].

James Greenwood and colleagues [25] provided a systematic review with meta-analysis in 2016 regarding rehabilitation after lumbar fusion. They concluded (with a total of 237 patients) that "complex rehabilitation" which included exercise and cognitive behavioral therapy offered short- and long-term benefits, decreasing disability and fear avoidance behavior, when compared to "usual care". As stated previously, cognitive behavioral education will likely be a large part of treatment, especially for patients requiring lumbar fusion. This review found that there is a high level of patient dissatisfaction following lumbar fusion, but cognitive behavioral treatment is directly linked to improved outcomes.

As a rehabilitation specialist, the other very important thing to keep in mind related to fusion is the change in mechanics that will occur because of the lack of mobility at one or more spinal segments. A spinal fusion literally means that that area of the spine no longer moves. Therefore, to get a functional level of mobility, the patient must move more above and below the level of fusion [12]. With the lumbar spine, that usually means the lower thoracic spine and, more importantly, the pelvis and hips.

As stated above, the complication that we need to be most aware of following lumbar fusion surgery is the possibility of future sacroiliac joint (SIJ) dysfunction. This occurs because of compensatory movement patterns at the pelvis due to lack of mobility of the lower lumbar spine. The SIJ is not designed to demonstrate large amounts of movement, and if the patient attempts to get movement here, they will likely strain and irritate ligaments around this joint. Instead, if the patient can be taught to move at the hips, the SIJ will be able to continue to provide stability at the pelvis, and the likelihood of SIJ injury is decreased.

Therefore, the therapist must start hip mobilization early in the rehabilitation process. Assessing for mobility restrictions of hip extension, and internal/external rotation during the initial evaluation will help guide treatment with the patient that can include stretching, hip joint mobilization, and SIJ stability exercises.

As with all rehabilitation patients, treatment should be guided by what is discovered during our evaluation. This will include the patient's specific goals, as well as objective impairments and functional limitations measured.

Intervention should focus on functional movements with an emphasis on keeping the spine in a neutral position and engaging the deep core musculature (multifidus and transverse abdominus). Instructing the patient in a neutral spine can be very difficult, especially for those patients with previous chronic low back pain and/or generalized pain. Specific neutral spine instruction is beyond the scope of this book, but we do provide some figures for reference (Figure 7.2).

The literature provides large amounts of research discussing the importance of therapeutic exercise as primary focus of plan of care [26, 27]. Yilmaz and colleagues[28] investigated the efficacy of a dynamic lumbar stabilization exercise program in patients with a recent lumbar microdiscectomy. The results of their randomized trial indicated that lumbar spinal stabilization exercises under the direction of a physical therapist were superior to performing a general exercise program independently at home and superior to a control group of no prescribed exercises at 3 months. The authors do caution that this study had a small sample size with 14 subjects in each group and did not describe any loss to follow-up.

Kulig et al. [29] performed a randomized clinical controlled trial comparing an intensive 12-week exercise program and education to education alone and usual physical therapy care following microdiscectomy. In the 2-group analyses, exercise and education resulted in a greater reduction in Oswestry Disability Index scores, and a greater improvement in distance walked compared to education alone. In the 3-group analyses, comparisons at the end of the program showed a significantly greater reduction in Oswestry Disability Index scores following exercise and education, compared with the education-only and usual physical therapy groups. The most recent clinical practice guideline reports that there is a need for high quality RCTs evaluating the effectiveness of different exercise training interventions for patients following surgery for LBP. "Clinicians should consider utilizing trunk coordination, strengthening, and endurance exercises to reduce low back pain and disability in patients with sub-acute and chronic low back pain with movement coordination impairments and in patients post lumbar microdiscectomy. (Recommendation based on strong evidence.)"

Patient education regarding movement patterns that limit compression, sheer or rotational forces will help patients see the connection between their pain and movement.

Depending on their fear of movement, Graded Exposure (Table 7.2) might be an important treatment strategy [30]. Compared to other lumbar surgeries, with microdiscectomy, soft tissue damage is minimal. However, pain, decreased mobility, and decreased trunk muscle strength can continue for months after surgery. This is likely due to lack of rehabilitation [31]. The most recent clinical practice guideline provides their recommendation regarding patient education during treatment. "Physical therapists may use general education (*i.e.*, postsurgical precautions, exercise, and resuming physical activity) for patients following lumbar spine surgery. This recommendation applies to those undergoing discectomy or decompression surgery." This is given with Level B evidence [5].

TAB. 7.2 Graded exposure.

	Session 1	Session 2	Session 3	Session 4
Fearful activity 1: Bending to lift object from ground				
Pre-activity fear level	50/100	50/100	60/100	50/100
Clinical activity	Supine knees to chest 2 min	Seated-knees to chest 2 min	Standing hip and knee flexion- neutral spine	Standing hip and knee flexion- mild lumbar flexion
Post-activity fear level	20/100	20/100	10/100	20/100
Fear reduced?	Yes	Yes	Yes	Yes
Plan	Progress to functional sitting	Progress to functional hip and knee hinge	Increase spine flexion movement	Increase duration of exercise

7.8 Postoperative Rehabilitation Protocols

This program is designed for those patients requiring extra assistance from a trained/certified physical therapist following more complicated surgical procedures and/or history of comorbidities.

Please note:

As each surgery is different and each patient is different, this plan is provided as a suggestion/guidance only. The program/plan is designed to be completed under the guidance of a rehabilitation specialist and should not be attempted independently, as it could lead to further injury.

See Table 7.3 for condensed version.

TAB. 7.3 Lumbar microdiscectomy treatment.

Phase 1 (Weeks 1–3): Protected Motion Phase
Patient Goals:
32. Manage edema and control pain with upright postures
33. Decrease associated fears
34. Good understanding of and use of proper body mechanics
35. Prevent adhesions that limit nerve mobility
36. Restore ROM and increase strength to lower extremities
37. Improve mobility of restricted joints

Patient Education:
38. Common to experience residual numbness following surgery – Likely to improve
39. Allow symptoms to guide activity
40. "Hurt does not equal harm"
41. Encourage to begin walking

Treatment:
Lower extremity passive ROM stretches
Dural/nerve glides/stretching in supine
Body mechanics training, walking program
Lower extremity training
Abdominal brace training

Milestones to Progress:
42. Adequate pain control during ADLs
43. Patient is able to maintain proper posture and positioning of spine during ADLs
44. No pain with abdominal bracing and isometric exercises

Phase 2 (Weeks 3–6): Progressive Loading/Strengthening
Goals:
45. Good neutral spine control in various positions
46. Continue increase lower extremity flexibility, strength
47. Minimal to no neural tension signs
48. Cardiovascular exercise 20 min
49. Decrease fear

Patient Education:
50. Progress walking tolerance as indicated
51. Continue to educate using pain neuroscience approach and Cognitive Behavioral Therapy

Treatment:
Progress neural mobilizations from gliders to tensioners
LE strengthening
Lifting instruction up to 2.5 kg
Progress abdominal brace training
Increase walking time and intensity

Milestones to Progress:
52. Adequate pain control during ADLs and physical activities
53. Can complete at least 20 min of aerobic activity
54. Demonstrates proper spinal positions and postures during therapeutic and aerobic exercises

TAB. 7.3 (continued).

Phase 3 (Weeks 7–12): Functional and Sensorimotor Training
Goals:
55. Consistent use of good body mechanics
56. Independent self-care and activities of daily living (ADL's)
57. Increase tolerance to physically demanding activities
58. Return to previous level of activity

Treatment:
Begin return to sport/work triplanar movement patterns
Progress core and LE strengthening in all planes of motion
Increase walking time and intensity

Milestones to Progress:
59. No pain during higher level function-specific activities
60. Demonstrates proper spinal postures and positions during higher level activities
61. Participating in an aerobic and strength training program to maintain fitness

Phase 4 (Weeks 12+): Sport/Work Specific Training
Treatment:
Progress full body strength and endurance
Incorporate jump and hop training (as appropriate)
Establish a walk/run independent program

Phase 1: Protected Motion Phase (Weeks 1–3)
Patient Goals:
1. Manage edema and control pain with upright postures
2. Decrease associated fears
3. Good understanding of and use of proper body mechanics
4. Prevent adhesions that limit nerve mobility
5. Restore range of motion (ROM) and increase strength to lower extremities
6. Improve mobility of restricted joints

Patient Education:

1. Common to experience residual numbness following surgery – Likely to improve
2. Allow symptoms to guide activity
3. "Hurt does not equal harm"
4. Encourage to begin walking

Treatment:

Passive ROM stretches
1. Hip flexion (knee bent), straight leg raise (SLR), hip external rotation stretch
2. Standing gastrocnemius-soleus stretch
Dural/nerve glides/stretching in supine (Figure 7.4)

Body mechanics training-

3. Bed mobility training

4. Maintain lumbar lordosis, avoid trunk flexion in sitting

Lower extremity training-

(2 × 20 repetitions to start 3 times a day):
1. Ankle pumps
2. Quad sets (tightening quadriceps muscle with leg straight) (Figure 7.5)
3. Long arc quadriceps (kicking leg straight in sitting)
4. Short arc quadriceps (straightening leg over pillow or foam roll)

Abdominal bracing-*(2 × 20 repetitions to start) 3 times a day:*
1. Abdominal isometrics (Figure 7.2)
2. Abdominal isometrics with hip abduction/external rotation (clams) (Figure 7.6)
3. Abdominal isometrics with hip abduction in hook-lying

Abdominal bracing progression-*(3 × 20 repetitions to start) 3 times a day:*
1. Abdominal isometric with heel slides
2. Abdominal isometric with upper extremity reach
3. Abdominal isometric with hip abduction in side-lying
4. Abdominal isometric with bridging (Figure 7.7)
5. Abdominal isometric with standing hip extension
6. Quadruped abdominal isometric, progressing to arm reach, leg reach, and alternating arm/leg reach (birddogs) (Figure 7.8)
7. Squatting (2–3 × 10 repetitions to start)

Walking Program

Milestones to Progress:
1. Adequate pain control during ADLs
2. Patient is able to maintain proper posture and positioning of spine during ADLs
3. No pain with abdominal bracing and isometric exercises

Phase 2: Progressive Loading/Strengthening (Week 3–6)

Goals:
1. Good neutral spine control in various positions
2. Continue to increase lower extremity flexibility, strength
3. Minimal to no neural tension signs
4. Cardiovascular exercise 20 minutes
5. Decrease fear

Patient Education:
1. Progress walking tolerance as indicated
2. Continue to educate using pain neuroscience approach and Cognitive Behavioral Therapy

Treatment:

LE strengthening
1. Squatting (2–3 × 10 repetitions to start)

Lifting instruction up to 2.5 kg (Figure 7.9)
Hip mobilization/stretching
Progress core control training:

1. Quadruped abdominal isometric, progressing to arm reach, leg reach, and alternating arm/leg reach (birddogs)
2. Prone hip extension (Figure 7.10)

Progress neural mobilizations from gliders to tensioners Figure 7.11
Increase walking time and intensity
Milestones to Progress:

1. Adequate pain control during ADLs and physical activities
2. Can complete at least 20 min of aerobic activity
3. Demonstrates proper spinal positions and postures during therapeutic and aerobic exercises

Phase 3: Functional and Sensorimotor Training (Weeks 7–12)
Goals:

1. Consistent use of good body mechanics
2. Independent self-care and activities of daily living (ADL's)
3. Increase tolerance to physically demanding activities
4. Return to previous level of activity

Treatment:
Begin return to sport/work triplanar movement patterns.
Progress core and LE strengthening in all planes of motion.

1. Front planks and side planks (Figure 7.12)
2. Squats while holding weight
3. Chopping/lifting exercise (Figure 7.13)

Increase walking time and intensity
Elliptical trainer
Milestones to Progress:

1. No pain during higher level function-specific activities
2. Demonstrates proper spinal postures and positions during higher level activities participating in an aerobic and strength training program to maintain fitness

Phase 4 Sport/Work Specific Training (Week 12+)
Treatment:
Progress full body strength and endurance

1. Squat and press
2. Turkish get-up Turkish

Incorporate jump and hop training (as appropriate) (Figure 7.14)
Establish a walk/run independent program

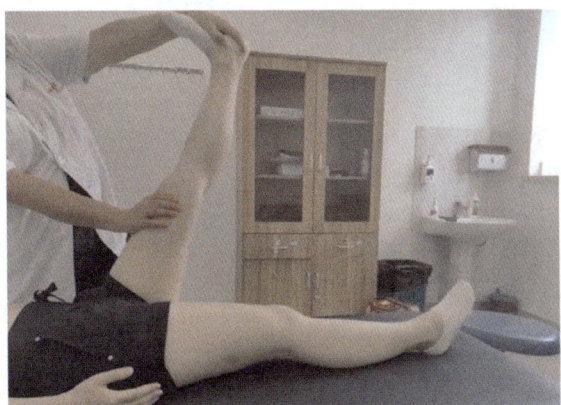

FIG. 7.4   Dural/nerve glides in supine.

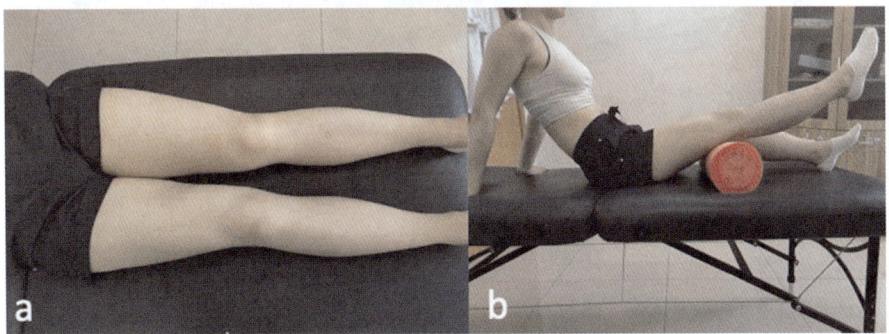

FIG. 7.5   Quad sets.
(a) isometric quadricep contraction; (b) Short arc quad.

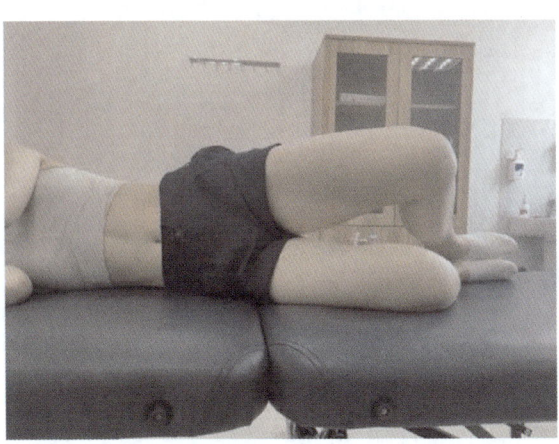

FIG. 7.6   Neutral spine with hip abduction/external rotation (also known as clams).

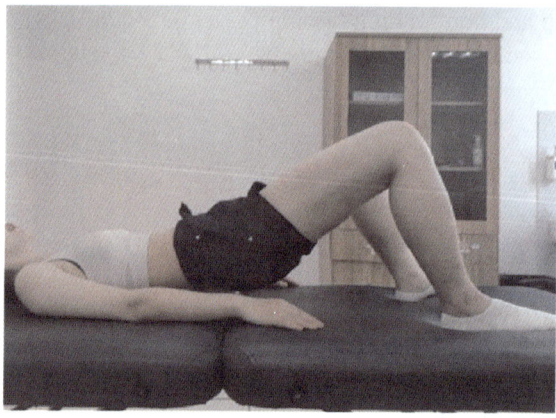

FIG. 7.7 Neutral spine with bridging.

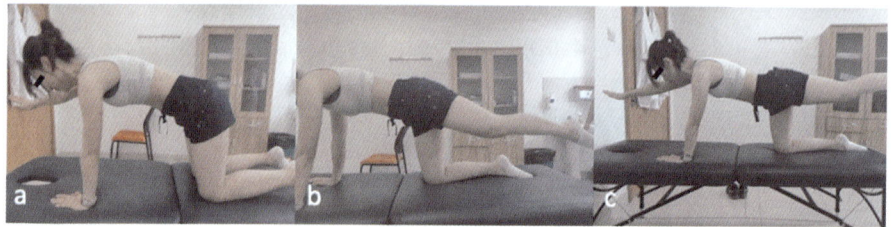

FIG. 7.8 Quadruped abdominal bracing progression.
(a) Quadruped neutral spine with arm reach; (b) Quadruped neutral spine with leg reach; (c) Quadruped neutral spine with alternating arm and leg reach (birddog).

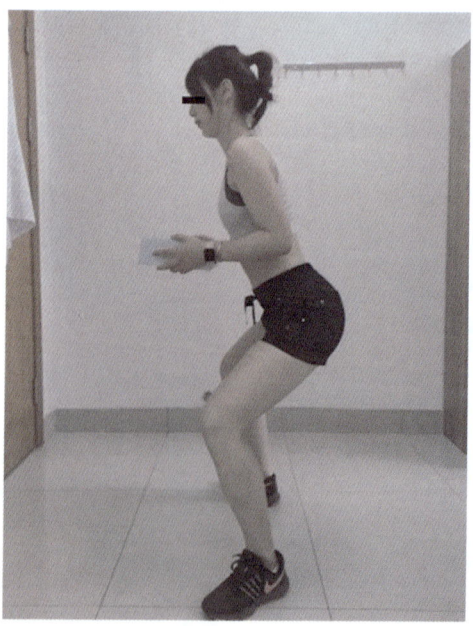

FIG. 7.9 Lifting instruction from low table, progressing to floor; lifting up to 2.5 kg.

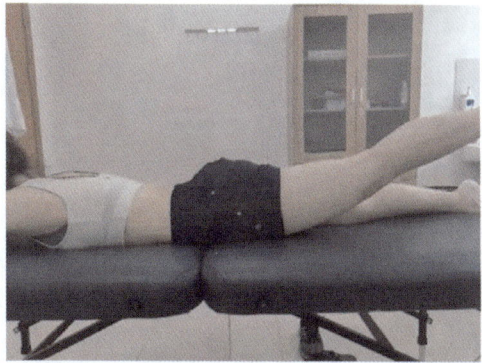

FIG. 7.10 Prone hip extension.

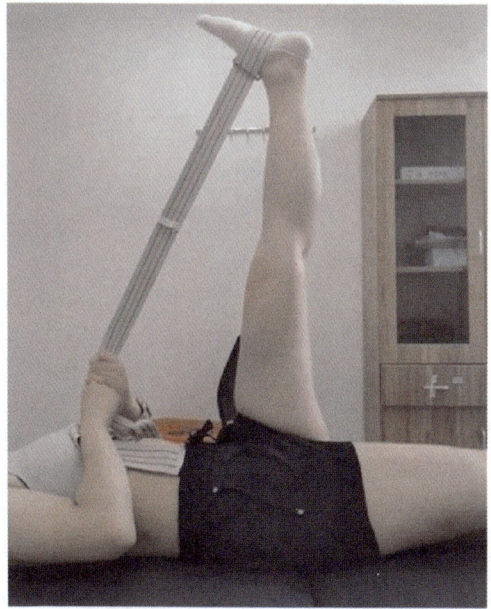

FIG. 7.11 Dural/nerve tensioning independently with belt.

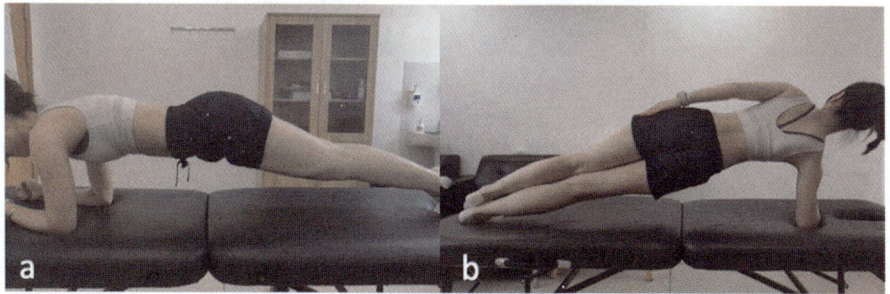

FIG. 7.12 Front and Side plank.
(a) Front plank; (b) Side plank.

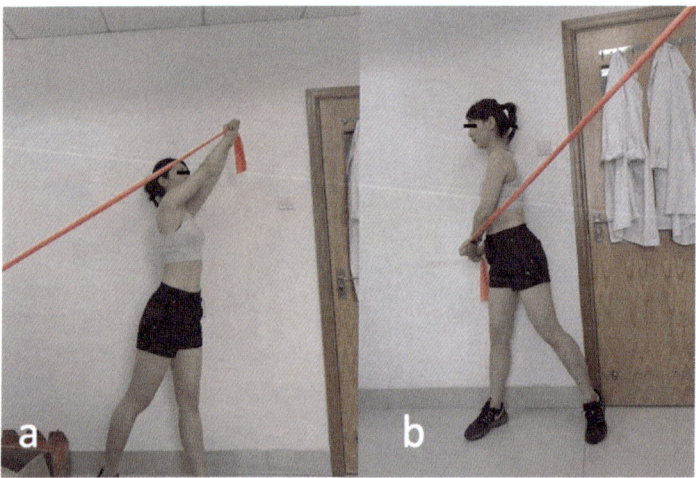

FIG. 7.13 Chopping/triplanar movements with resistance

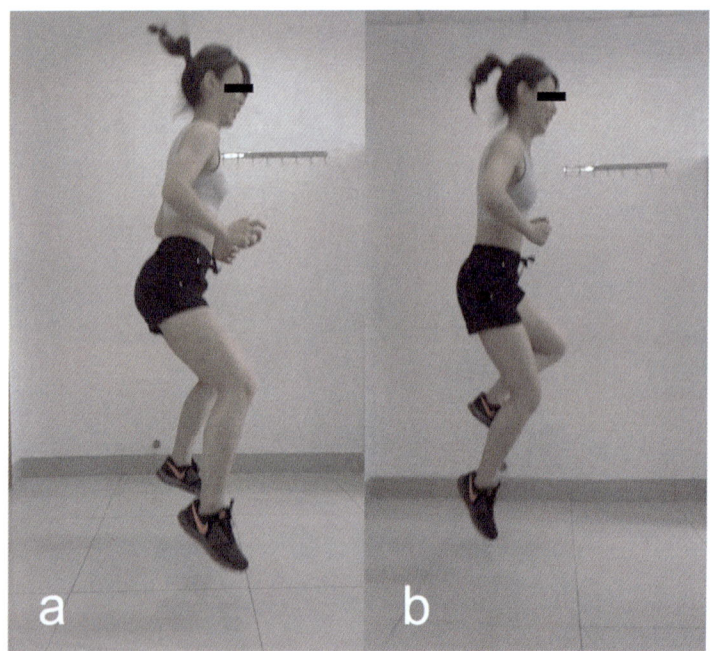

FIG. 7.14 Jump and hop training.
(a) Jumping training; (b) Hopping training.

Lumbar Fusion Rehabilitation Treatment Protocol

This program is designed for those patients requiring extra assistance from a trained/ certified physical therapist following more complicated surgical procedures and/or history of comorbidities.

Please note:

As each surgery is different and each patient is different, this plan is provided as a suggestion/guidance only. The program/plan is designed to be completed under the guidance of a rehabilitation specialist and should not be attempted independently, as it could lead to further injury.

See Table 7.4 for condensed version.

TAB. 7.4   Lumbar fusion treatment.

Phase 1 (Weeks 1–2): Protected Motion Phase
Patient Goals:
62. Control pain and inflammation
63. Protect repair
64. Teach proper alignment through positioning and controlled movement
65. No evidence of fear-avoidance

Patient Education:
1. Common to experience residual numbness following surgery – Likely to improve
2. Allow symptoms to guide activity
3. "Hurt does not equal harm"
4. Encourage to begin walking

Treatment:
Cognitive behavioral therapy/education
TLSO brace to limit lumbar motion
Perform controlled mobility with neutral spine precautions
Walk as much as tolerated
Bed level exercises/lower extremity training

Milestones to Progress:
1. Adequate pain control during ADLs
2. Can don/doff TLSO brace with independence
3. Performs bed mobility with proper posture and no pain

Phase 2 (Weeks 3–6): Progressive Loading/Strengthening
Goals:
4. Pain and inflammation control
5. Kinesthetic training for maintaining neutral spine
6. Activation of transverse abdominus & multifidus
7. Proper body mechanics with all functional activities
8. Improve flexibility of hip region

Patient Education:
1. Altered lumbar and pelvic coordination common with low back pain, especially with forward bending, rising from chair and walking
2. Lifting instruction up to 2.5 kg/5 lbs
3. Encourage walking as much as possible
4. Continue to educate using pain neuroscience approach and Cognitive Behavioral Therapy

Treatment:
Ice, electrical stimulation, STM (if indicated)
Education & practice of maintaining a neutral spine posture
Dynamic lumbar stabilization exercises in neutral spine
LE strengthening
Hip flexor and rotator stretches

TAB. 7.4 (continued).

Functional activity training in proper alignment
Milestones to Progress:
1. Adequate pain control during ADLs and physical activities
2. Can complete at least 20 min of aerobic activity
3. Demonstrates proper spinal positions and postures during therapeutic and aerobic exercises

Phase 3 (Weeks 7–16): Functional and Sensorimotor Training
Goals:
1. Automatic activation of deep core musculature
2. Progress dynamic lumbar stabilization
3. Progress aerobic activity
4. Improve tolerance and confidence with forward bending
5. Sport simulation/controlled environment

Treatment:
Functional training with focus on forward bend, sit-to-stand (work conditioning if appropriate)
Aerobic exercises
Begin return to sport/work triplanar movement patterns
Progress core and LE strengthening in all planes of motion
Increase walking time and intensity

Milestones to Progress:
1. No pain during higher level function-specific activities
2. Confidence with forward bending
3. Demonstrates proper spinal postures and positions during higher level activities
4. Participating in an aerobic and strength training program to maintain fitness

Phase 4 (Weeks 16+): Sport/Work Specific Training
Treatment:
Progress full body strength and endurance
Incorporate jump and hop training (as appropriate)
Establish a walk/run independent program

Phase 1: Protected Motion Phase (Weeks 1–2)
Patient Goals:

1. Control pain and inflammation
2. Protect repair
3. Teach proper alignment through positioning and controlled movement
4. No evidence of fear-avoidance

Patient Education:

5. Common to experience residual numbness following surgery – Likely to improve
6. Allow symptoms to guide activity
7. "Hurt does not equal harm"

8. Encourage to begin walking

Treatment:

1. Cognitive behavioral therapy/education
2. TLSO brace to limit lumbar motion
3. Perform controlled mobility with neutral spine precautions
4. Walk as much as tolerated
5. Bed level exercises:

(1) Quad sets, glut sets, heel slides, heel raises, etc.
Passive ROM stretches
(2) Hip flexion (knee bent), straight leg raise (SLR), hip external rotation stretch
(3) Standing gastrocnemius-soleus stretch

Dural/nerve glides/stretching in supine
Body mechanics training-

(4) Bed mobility training
(5) Maintain lumbar lordosis, avoid trunk flexion in sitting

Lower extremity training-
(2 × 20 repetitions to start 3 times a day):

6. Ankle pumps
7. Quad sets (tightening quadriceps muscle with leg straight)
8. Long arc quadriceps (kicking leg straight in sitting)
9. Short arc quadriceps (straightening leg over pillow or foam roll)

Abdominal bracing-*(2 × 20 repetitions to start) 3 times a day:*

10. Abdominal isometrics
11. Abdominal isometrics with hip abduction/external rotation (clams)
12. Abdominal isometrics with hip abduction in hook-lying

Walking Program
Milestones to Progress:

13. Adequate pain control during ADLs
14. Can don/doff TLSO brace with independence
15. Performs bed mobility with proper posture and no pain

Phase 2: Progressive Loading/Strengthening (Week 3–6)
Goals:

1. Pain and inflammation control
2. Kinesthetic training for maintaining neutral spine
3. Activation of transverse abdominus & multifidus
4. Proper body mechanics with all functional activities
5. Improve flexibility of hip region

Patient Education:

1. Altered lumbar and pelvic coordination common with low back pain, especially with forward bending, rising from chair, and walking
2. Lifting instruction up to 2.5 kg/5 lbs
3. Encourage walking as much as possible
4. Continue to educate using pain neuroscience approach and Cognitive Behavioral Therapy

Treatment:
Ice, electrical stimulation, STM (if indicated)
Education & practice of maintaining a neutral spine posture
Hip flexor and rotator stretches
Functional activity training in proper alignment
LE strengthening

5. Squatting (2–3 × 10 repetitions to start)

Lifting instruction up to 2.5 kg
Progress core control training:
Abdominal bracing progression-*(3 × 20 repetitions to start) 3 times a day:*

6. Abdominal isometric with heel slides
7. Abdominal isometric with upper extremity reach
8. Abdominal isometric with hip abduction in side-lying
9. Abdominal isometric with bridging
10. Abdominal isometric with standing hip extension
11. Quadruped abdominal isometric, progressing to arm reach, leg reach, and alternating arm/leg reach (birddogs)
12. Squatting (2–3 × 10 repetitions to start)
13. Prone hip extension

Progress neural mobilizations from gliders to tensioners
Increase walking time and intensity

Milestones to Progress:

14. Adequate pain control during ADLs and physical activities
15. Can complete at least 20 min of aerobic activity
16. Demonstrates proper spinal positions and postures during therapeutic and aerobic exercises

Phase 3: Functional and Sensorimotor Training (Weeks 7–16)
Goals:

1. Automatic activation of deep core musculature
2. Progress dynamic lumbar stabilization
3. Progress aerobic activity
4. Improve tolerance and confidence with forward bending
5. Sport simulation/controlled environment

Treatment:
Trunk strengthening exercises
Front/side planks, anti-rotational wood chops
Extremity strengthening
Functional training with focus on forward bend, sit-to-stand (work conditioning if appropriate)
Aerobic exercises
Walking, dancing, elliptical, bicycle, swimming
Begin return to sport/work triplanar movement patterns.
Progress core and LE strengthening in all planes of motion.

6. Front planks and side planks
7. Squats while holding weight
8. Chopping/lifting exercise

Increase walking time and intensity
Elliptical trainer

Milestones to Progress:

9. No pain during higher level function-specific activities
10. Confidence with forward bending
11. Demonstrates proper spinal postures and positions during higher level activities
12. Participating in an aerobic and strength training program to maintain fitness

Phase 4: Sport/Work Specific Training (Week 16+)
Treatment:
Progress full body strength and endurance

1. Squat and press
2. Turkish get-up Turkish

Incorporate jump and hop training (as appropriate)
Establish a walk/run independent program

References

[1] Hoy D., March L., Brooks P., *et al.* (2014) The global burden of low back pain: Estimates from the Global Burden of Disease 2010 study, *Ann. Rheum. Dis.* **73**, 968.
[2] Meucci R.D., Fassa A.G., Faria N.M. (2015) Prevalence of chronic low back pain: Systematic review, *Rev. Saude Publica* **49**, 1.
[3] Cawley D., Alexander M., Morris S. (2014) Multifidus innervation and muscle assessment post-spinal surgery, *Eur. Spine J.* **23**, 320.
[4] Delitto A., *et al.* (2012) Low back pain, *JOSPT*.
[5] George S., *et al.* (2021) Physical therapist interventions for low back pain: Low back pain revision 2021, *JOSPT*.
[6] Madera M., *et al.* (2017) The role of physical therapy and rehabilitation after lumbar fusion surgery for degenerative disease: A systematic review, *J. Neurosurg. Spine* **26**, 694.
[7] Rowley K.M., Smith J.A., Kulig K. (2019) Reduced trunk coupling in persons with recurrent low back pain is associated with greater deep-to-superficial trunk muscle activation ratios

during the balance-dexterity task, *JOSPT* **49**, 887.
[8] Sions J.M., Elliot J.M., Pohlig R., Hicks G. (2017) Trunk muscle characteristics of the multifidi, erector spinae, psoas, and quadratus lumborum in older adults with and without chronic low back pain, *JOSPT* **47**, 173.
[9] Hodges P., et al. (2015) Mulitifidus muscle changes after back surgery are characterized by structural remodeling of muscle, adipose and connective tissue, not muscle atrophy, *Spine* **40**, 1057.
[10] Hodges P., Danneels L. (2019) Changes in structure and function of the back muscles in low back pain: Different time points, observations and mechanisms, *JOSPT* **49**, 464.
[11] Hodges P., et al. (2019) Diverse role of biological plasticity in low back pain and its impact on sensorimotor control of the spine, *JOSPT* **49**, 389.
[12] Pao J.-L., et al. (2014) Trunk control ability after minimally invasive lumbar fusion surgery during the early postoperative phase, *J. Phys. Ther. Sci.* **26**, 1165.
[13] Tarnanen S., et al. (2018) Neutral spine control exercises in rehabilitation after lumbar spine fusion, *J. Strength Cond. Res.* **28**, 2018.
[14] Louw A., Butler D.S., Diener I., Puentedura E.J. (2013) Development of a preoperative neuroscience educational program for patients with lumbar radiculopathy, *Am. J. Phys. Med. Rehabil.* **92**(5), 446.
[15] Ojha H., et al. (2016) Timing of physical therapy initiation for nonsurgical management of musculoskeletal disorders and effects on patient outcomes: A systematic review, *JOSPT* **46**, 56.
[16] Shriver M., et al. (2015) Lumbar microdiscectomy complication rates: A systematic review and meta-analysis, *Neurosurg. Focus* **39**, E6.
[17] Chen Y.-C., et al. (2019) An updated meta-analysis of clinical outcomes comparing minimally invasive with open transforaminal lumbar interbody fusion in patients with degenerative lumbar diseases, *Medicine* **98**, 43.
[18] Dayani F., et al. (2018) Minimally invasive lumbar pedicle screw fixation using cortical bone trajectory-screw accuracy, complications, and learning curve in 100 screw placements, *J. Clin. Neurosci.*
[19] Chen X., et al. (2020) Complication rates of different discectomy techniques for symptomatic lumbar disc herniation: A systematic review and meta-analysis, *Eur. Spine J.*
[20] Clark A., et al. (2017) Tubular microdiscectomy: Techniques, complication avoidance and review of literature, *Neurosurg. Focus* **43**, E7.
[21] Norton B.J., Sahrmann S.A., Van Dillen L.R. (2004) Differences in measurements of lumbar curvature related to gender and low back pain, *JOSPT* **34**, 524.
[22] Oestergaard L., et al. (2013) Early versus late initiation of rehabilitation after lumbar spine fusion, *Spine* **38**, 1979.
[23] Oosterhuis T., et al. (2014) Rehabilitation after lumbar disc surgery, *Cochrane Database Syst. Rev.* **3**, CD003007.
[24] Ozkara G.O., et al. (2015) Effectiveness of physical therapy and rehabilitation programs starting immediately after lumbar disc surgery, *Turk Neurosurg.* **3**, 372.
[25] Greenwood J., et al. (2016) Rehabilitation following lumbar fusion surgery: A systematic review and meta-analysis, *Spine* **41**, E28.
[26] Dolan P., Greenfield K., Nelson R.J., Nelson I.W. (2000) Can exercise therapy improve the outcome of microdiscectomy? *Spine* **25**(12), 1523.
[27] Ostelo R.W., Costa L.O., Maher C.G., de Vet H.C., van Tulder M.W. (2004) Rehabilitation after lumbar disc surgery, *Cochrane Data-base Syst. Rev.* **4**, CD003007.
[28] Yilmaz F., et al. (2003) Efficacy of dynamic lumbar stabilization exercises in lumbar microdiscectomy, *J. Rehabil. Med.* **35**, 163.
[29] Kulig K., et al. (2009) An intensive, progressive exercise program reduces disability and improves functional performance in patients after single-level lumbar microdiscectomy, *Phys. Ther.* **89**, 1145.
[30] George S., Zeppieri G. (2009) Physical therapy utilization of graded exposure in patients with low back pain, *JOSPT* **39**, 496.
[31] Hakkinen A., Ylinen J., Kautiainen H., et al. (2003) Pain, trunk muscle strength, spine mobility and disability following lumbar disc surgery, *J. Rehabil. Med.* **35**, 236.